THE EAT-CLEAN DIET® Stripped

Peel Off Those Last 10 Pounds!

NEW YORK TIMES BEST-SELLING AUTHOR

TOSCA RENO

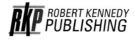

RKP ROBERT KENNEDY PUBLISHING

Published by
Robert Kennedy Publishing
400 Matheson Blvd. West
Mississauga, ON
L5R 3M1 Canada

Visit us at **www.eatcleandiet.com**,
www.rkpubs.com and **www.toscareno.com**

Library and Archives Canada Cataloguing
in Publication

Reno, Tosca, 1959-
        The eat-clean diet stripped : peel off
those last 10 pounds / Tosca Reno.

Includes index.
ISBN 978-1-55210-086-8

        1. Reducing diets. 2. Weight loss. I.
Title.

RM222.2.R4648 2011   613.2'5
C2010-906763-0

10 9 8 7 6 5 4 3 2 1

Distributed in Canada by
NBN (National Book Network)
67 Mowat Avenue, Suite 241
Toronto, ON
M6K 3E3

Distributed in USA by
NBN (National Book Network)
15200 NBN Way
Blue Ridge Summit, PA
17214

Printed in Canada

Robert Kennedy Publishing
BOOK DEPARTMENT

MANAGING DIRECTOR
Wendy Morley

MANAGING ONLINE EDITOR
Vinita Persaud

PRODUCTION EDITOR
Cali Hoffman

**ONLINE EDITOR & EDITORIAL
ASSISTANT**
Meredith Barrett

ASSOCIATE EDITOR
Rachel Corradetti

ONLINE EDITOR
Kiersten Corradetti

EDITORIAL ASSISTANTS
Tara Kher, Sharlene Liladhar

ONLINE ASSISTANT
Chelsea Kennedy

ART DIRECTOR
Gabriella Caruso Marques

ASSISTANT ART DIRECTOR
Jessica Pensabene Hearn

EDITORIAL DESIGNERS
Brian Ross, Ellie Jeon

ART ASSISTANT
Kelsey-Lynn Corradetti

RECIPE DEVELOPER
Kierstin Buchner
www.kierstinbuchner.com

RECIPE PHOTOS
Photographer– **Donna Griffith**
www.donnagriffith.com
Food Stylist– **Claire Stubbs**

INDEXING AND PROOFREADING
James De Medeiros

IMPORTANT

The information in this book reflects the author's
experiences and opinions and is not intended to
replace medical advice.

Before beginning this or any nutritional or exercise
regimen, consult your physician to be sure it is
appropriate for you. Ask for a physical stress test.

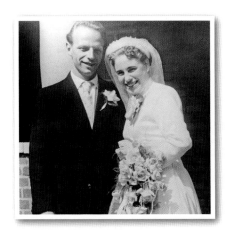

To my very fit mother, Tina,
and my beloved father, Bill,
who is no longer with us.

contents

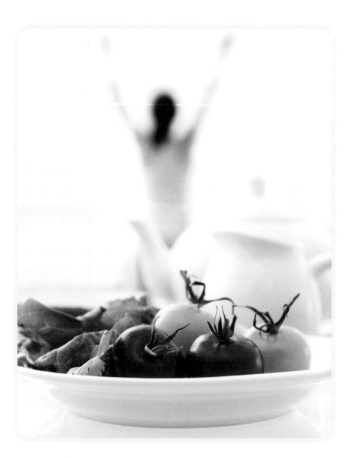

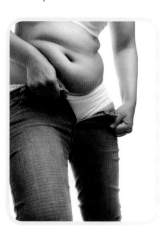

"We have to trick our bodies into letting go of those last 10 pounds."

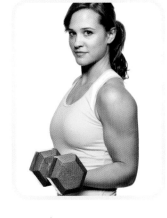

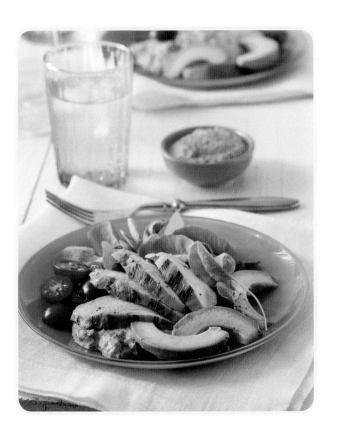

Introduction

The average woman wants to lose 10 pounds, and with good reason – those last pounds hold on tight! If you work out regularly and eat right, or if you don't really take great care of yourself but don't overeat, or even if you've lost a lot of weight already, you probably want to lose about 10 pounds. Our bodies hang on to those last few because we are genetically programmed that way. When our body-fat level drops below a certain point, our bodies cling to every ounce to protect us from starving. In order to get rid of the last 10 pounds, we have to find ways to trick our bodies into dropping fat.

Lucky for us, physique competitors have worked it all out. Every year – sometimes two or three times a year – these competitors gain weight while building up their muscles, and then they must drop that excess fat in order to show their physiques to full magnificence. With a tough schedule like that, and knowing they will be standing onstage in next-to-nothing in front of judges ... well, they leave nothing to chance.

But you don't have to be a competitor to benefit from their knowledge. There are lots of reasons you might want to lose 10 pounds. You might be going on a beach vacation and want to look

"This entire book is dedicated to you, the person who doesn't have a whole lot of weight to lose and doesn't want to go on a 'diet,' but wants to take her body to the next level."

great in a bikini, or maybe you're getting married and want to be the most beautiful bride you can be, or perhaps you have a high school reunion and want to show your ex-boyfriend what a huge mistake he made. You may have no overwhelming reason, but just want to look and feel your best. Whatever the reason, I know you want to lose them because you're holding this book in your hands!

This entire book is dedicated to you, the person who doesn't have a whole lot of weight to lose and doesn't want to go on a "diet," but wants to take her body to the next level. This book is about using diet and exercise to trick your metabolism into letting you drop those final 10 pounds. It's about using specific herbs and other food items to work in your favor. This book offers tricks of the fitness pros, tips on getting rid of cellulite, and lots of motivation – so you will allow yourself to finally succeed. In short, this book offers everything you need to reach your goal – so take the leap! What have you got to lose? Nothing but those last 10 pounds.

Sincerely,

Tosca Reno

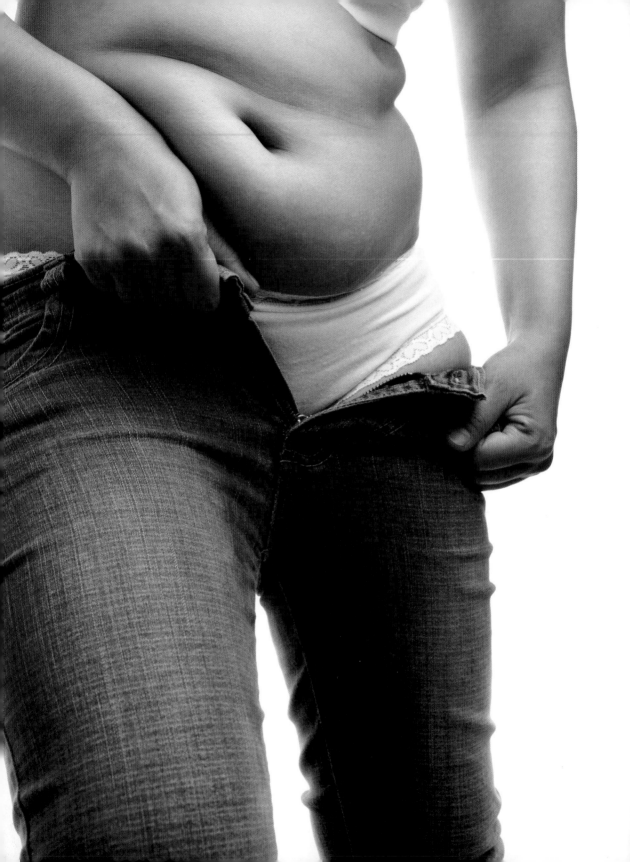

1 | Does an Extra 10 Pounds of Fat Really Matter?

The entire objective of this book, *The Eat-Clean Diet Stripped*, is to help you get rid of those last 10 pounds of excess weight, fast. These final pounds seem to be the most difficult and the most irritating to shed for the vast majority of us. I know from personal experience that the last 10 pounds are the ones that require a little extra push from you in just about everything you do, from eating to training to cleansing. I intend to help you do just that.

> ## "People struggle with those last 10 for many reasons."

Who's Thinking of Losing Weight?

In North America, 67 percent of our population is overweight, and according to the World Health Organization (WHO), obesity has reached epidemic numbers. Apparently millions, if not billions, of us around the world are thinking of losing weight, whether 10 pounds or 110 pounds. Few are exempt from this problem. The population of overweight children is larger than ever, not only in North America, where the number of overweight children has doubled since 1980, but also worldwide, where the WHO estimates that 17.6 million children under the age of five are overweight. In America alone, 200 million individuals are overweight or obese.

Stepping away from statistics for a moment, let's consider why you might be interested in shedding those annoying last 10 pounds. Throughout your life will be moments when you want to look your best. You may simply decide on a haircut and a new dress, or you might look in the mirror and realize your waistline needs trimming. Frowning, you look at the calendar and realize you have only 28 days until your wedding day, your son's bar mitzvah or your beach vacation. I've certainly found myself in a similar situation.

People struggle with those last 10 for many reasons. Perhaps you have already lost a considerable amount of weight but have hit a plateau. Somehow those final pounds are clinging furiously to your midsection. Or maybe you must lose weight to prepare for an operation. Doctors often postpone surgery until their patient reaches a size that decreases the risks. I know of a gentleman who had to undergo prostate surgery and was told to lose 10 pounds before the doc would even consider it. The poor fellow had to endure his embarrassing symptoms for another few weeks before he could get relief.

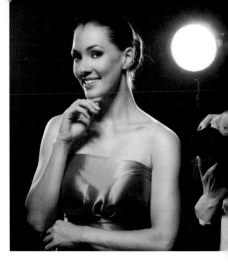

▲ **LOOK AND FEEL** your absolute best at a big event.

Hundreds of people, from the bride-to-be to the newly single, are looking for a surefire method to drop 10 pounds in a hurry. The good news is that you can – and will – do it. Remember when the tabloids reported that Jessica Simpson lost 10 pounds in two weeks? That was probably an exaggeration to sell magazines and let's be serious, 10 pounds in two weeks? I don't think so! I think she just had bad styling advice when she wore those "mom jeans" on stage, but even celebrities sometimes need to strip off excess weight fast. If I were a celeb attending the Oscars, I would definitely be thinking of ways to tighten up in time for the big event. A few pounds can make the difference between boring and fantastic, the latter landing you in the pages of *InStyle* magazine strutting your hottest Oscar look ... hey, a girl can dream!

So There You Are and Here We Go!

Let this be the start of stripping away those final 10 pounds forever. Take heart that *The Eat-Clean Diet Stripped* will serve as your no-fail guide to get the job done. Loads of people are in the same boat looking for just this kind of help. Relying on the Eat-Clean Diet Principles along with some secrets I have learned from those in the business of shaping razor-sharp physiques plus a few more tips and tricks, you will soon lose those last few for good!

I can guarantee you will experience success because I already know how well *The Eat-Clean Diet* works not just for me, but for hundreds of thousands of others. I lost the weight that had been clinging to me 10 years ago by following the Eat-Clean Diet Principles and learning to train with weights, as have many others, according to the success stories that pour in daily. People who discover the Eat-Clean Diet lifestyle transform their lives from sick and sedentary to robust and raring to go. We know Eating Clean works.

"Loads of people are in the same boat looking for just this kind of help."

> "I have no desire to look like a She-Man. I love being a woman and I intend to keep it that way."

It still amazes me that life can be changed so profoundly – either for better or worse – just by making food choices. I love that I look and feel better now than I did in my 30s. I feel as if I am harboring a guilty secret from others because I don't look or feel tired or aging even though I am in my 50s.

Physique Athletes: Our Teachers

I am going to share the secrets of physique athletes with you. These are the people who taught me everything I know about Clean food, weight training and shedding the last 10 pounds fast. I'm going to give you so many tricks and tips from the industry, you may not be prepared for the wonderful changes about to take place!

Who are physique athletes? When you flip open a copy of *Shape*, *Women's Health* or *Oxygen* magazine, the women you see are physique athletes. When you attend a fitness, figure or bikini contest, the competitors are physique athletes. Even women who compete in bodybuilding are considered physique athletes. I am also a physique athlete since I have competed several times in bodybuilding, figure and bikini competitions. Many envy these women who have not a pound of excess fat, have tight waistlines and look confident, happy and radiant.

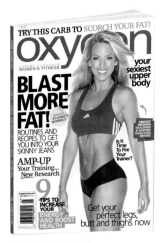

▲ **THE WOMEN** on the cover of *Oxygen* magazine keep their figures tight by following the *Eat-Clean Diet* Principles.

Rachel McLish (right) has inspired me the most with her long, lean and fluid muscular lines. When I began to transform my physique I would often look at pictures of Rachel McLish to keep myself inspired. I have no desire to look like a She-Man. I love being a woman and I intend to keep it that way, and Rachel's body looked like the one I wanted to have. The physiques of Monica Brant and Jamie Eason also inspire me because these are examples of women who labor at shaping a stellar, muscular yet beautiful body. They are beautiful and shapely through the efforts of their own hard work.

It was my preparation for physique competitions that taught me much of what I know and do today to help people Clean up their eating and training lifestyles. The preparation for each contest is grueling, long, lonely and challenging, but this is where I learned so many of the slimming tricks I will be sharing with you in this book. When your career depends on owning a lean and noteworthy physique, you had better know how to keep it tight and toned. I don't think anyone but a physique athlete could provide such sound and effective advice. Think about it – a physique athlete has to get up on

"It was my preparation for physique competitions that taught me much of what I know and do today."

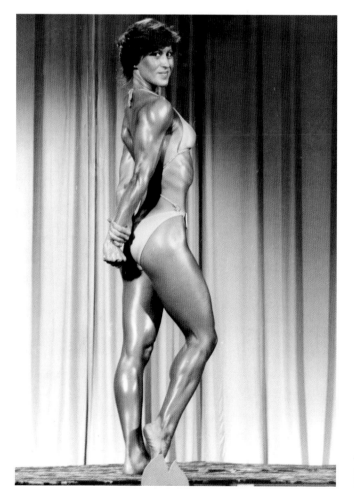

◄ QUEEN OF BODYBUILDING
Rachel McLish poses at her 1980 Ms. Olympia victory.

"Nutrition —
the food we
eat every day
— decides
how we look
and feel."

stage wearing little more than a teeny-tiny swimsuit, strut her stuff and then let the judges and everyone else in the audience analyze her goods. There is no more intense scrutiny than this. A contestant will have used every trick she knows to get herself lean and tight to prepare for this moment. Now you are going to learn these tricks too.

Body Beautiful / Body Healthy

Often a competitor's success comes down to whether or not she has been able to get lean enough for contest day. This involves weeks and weeks of preparation, including dieting and weight training. The diet tricks are the ones we will focus on the most, as it is predominantly the food we eat that shapes how we look. As our late friend fitness guru Jack LaLanne says in his book, *Live Young Forever*, "Eating Clean is the only way to lose unwanted fat."

In each of the *Eat-Clean Diet* books I have written, I spend a little time explaining how to approach the renovation of your physique. There are three significant factors involved in the effort to lose weight and sculpt a lean physique. These include: nutrition, training and genetics.

As we consider these three factors (nutrition, training and genetics), I want to place them in the correct balance so you will know where to direct your energy as you begin your own physique transformation. Most people think training does the lion's share of the job, but in reality nutrition – the food we eat every day – decides how we look and feel. That can go either way of course. If you eat a lot of greasy, processed, "anti" food you will look greasy, gray and dead. On the other hand if you eat wholesome, Clean foods you will look vibrant, radiant and slim. Finally, genetics affect your looks. There is little anyone can do about the width of their hip bones or length of their torso. I like to put the three factors

BODY BEAUTIFUL / BODY HEALTHY FORMULA

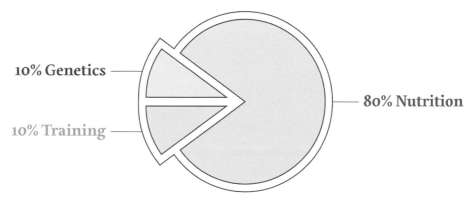

10% Genetics ———

10% Training ———

——— **80% Nutrition**

80% Nutrition + 10% Training + 10% Genetics =
Body Beautiful / Body Healthy

---

into a formula I call the Body Beautiful / Body Healthy formula.

80% Nutrition + 10% Training + 10% Genetics =
Body Beautiful / Body Healthy

Once you understand how critical your food choices are in relation to your efforts to strip your body of unwanted fat, you may think twice about eating that Twinkie. Instead you will eat foods that contribute to building a better you. These foods are called Clean foods and are stripped bare of non-essential elements. What you eat from here on in is a critical key to your weight-loss success. You are going to love the changes about to happen to your body.

How Does An Extra 10 Pounds Affect Your Health?

Whether or not you have accepted the added weight on your frame, I can guarantee your body hasn't. Extra caloric intake wreaks havoc on your system. Aside from the unappealing nature of rolls of fat under your skin, have you ever considered the array of damage that extra fat is doing to the parts of you that you can't see? If you

> "If you eat wholesome, Clean foods you will look vibrant, radiant and slim."

"With over 300,000 deaths related to obesity each year, it's time to get serious about your health and not just your skinny jeans!"

haven't considered this before, let me be the first to inform you of the numerous health risks linked to your added weight. Even a small increase in weight (10 to 20 pounds) can lead to increased risk of death. With over 300,000 deaths related to obesity each year, it's time to get serious about your health and not just your skinny jeans!

The Top 10 Health Risks Caused By Your Added 10

1 Type 2 Diabetes

With extra fat on your frame, your body has difficulty handling post-meal blood-sugar loads. Your body becomes resistant to insulin, the hormone responsible for controlling your blood-sugar levels. Excess fat also kills off the cells that produce insulin. Both of these put you at major risk for developing type 2 diabetes. The Office of the Surgeon General tells us that almost 90 percent of individuals with type 2 diabetes are overweight, and a weight gain of only 11 to 18 pounds doubles your risk of developing this disorder. Studies have shown that losing five to seven percent of your body weight will vastly improve your health and reduce your chances of developing type 2 diabetes. With 21 million Americans already suffering from this disorder, according to the American Diabetes Association, there's no time like the present to lose the fat and cut your risk.

2 Heart & Cerebrovascular Disease

Extra lipids (a fancy word for fat) in your diet elevate your risk of heart attack and stroke. When you carry excess fat, low-density lipoprotein (LDL) values increase, while high-density lipoprotein (HDL) values decrease. When this ratio is thrown off HDL can no longer remove enough excess cholesterol from your bloodstream and plaque formations develop in your arteries. Plaque-coated arteries cause the heart to work much harder to

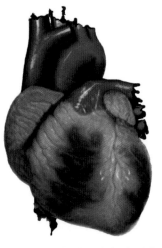

▲ **HEART DISEASE** is the leading killer of North Americans.

push blood through the body, consequently causing an increase in blood pressure, enlarged heart size, and thrombus formations around the plaques. Ultimately, heart and cerebrovascular disease develop increasing the risk of experiencing a heart attack or stroke. For every five extra pounds of fat you carry on your frame, your body creates three more miles of blood vessels. Just imagine the strain this puts on your heart! Lose the weight and lose the risk.

"Keep this muscle beating strong by losing the weight and the risk."

3 Metabolic Syndrome

Metabolic syndrome is a collection of disorders that increase your chance of developing diabetes and cardiovascular disease. Weight gain increases blood pressure and LDL, and decreases HDL and insulin resistance. This is especially true for anyone carrying excess belly fat. Statistics from the American Heart Association show that 35 percent of men and 33 percent of women suffer from this condition in the United States. Simply reducing your portion sizes and processed food intake, along with increasing your fruit and vegetable intake and activity level, put you at a much lower risk of acquiring metabolic syndrome.

4 Cancer

The "C" word has become one of the most dreaded conditions of our time, and excess fat is a risk factor. While the direct link between cancer and extra pounds has yet to be officially determined, the theory is that fat cells release hormones that encourage unregulated growth of tumor cells while also putting your body in a constant state of inflammation. According to a study conducted by the *Annals of Internal Medicine*, overweight men have a greater chance of developing colorectal and prostate cancer, while overweight women have a greater risk of developing cancer of the endometrium, gallbladder, cervix, ovary and breast. The Office of the Surgeon General tells us that middle-

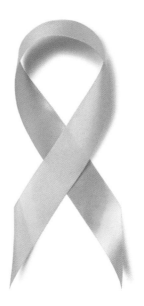

▲ **MAINTAINING** a healthy weight and eating a diet rich in fruits and vegetables is the best preventative medicine.

> "Being overweight means you are at risk of developing depression, and being depressed puts you at a greater risk of being overweight."

aged women who have gained more than 20 pounds since the age of 18 increase their risk of developing postmenopausal breast cancer twofold. A loss of even 10 pounds can greatly reduce your risk of developing cancer. I believe eating vegetables and fruit are much more appealing than chemotherapy.

5 Musculoskeletal Issues

Weight gain means body strains! Carrying around extra weight increases the wear and tear on your joints. Studies conducted by the National Institute of Health suggest that added weight causes musculoskeletal discomfort in people of all ages, even adolescents, who put themselves at a greater risk for fractures. This discomfort continues into adulthood, when overweight individuals are at a greater risk of developing osteoarthritis, and in worst-case scenarios need full knee and hip replacements. Arthritis also becomes increasingly prevalent in overweight individuals because of the inflammatory nature of fat cell products, which increase swelling and discomfort in joints. The Johns Hopkins Arthritis Center warns us that a weight gain of only 10 pounds increases the force placed on each knee with each step by 30 to 60 pounds, while the Office of the Surgeon General claims that a weight gain of as little as two pounds increases the risk of developing arthritis by nine to 13 percent. Ouch! We've only got one set of joints, so let's keep them healthy and happy with regular exercise and a Clean diet.

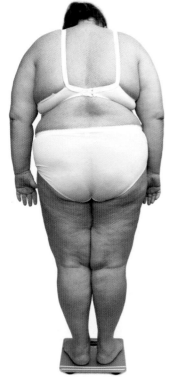

6 Depression

Both the chemical and physical side effects of increased weight can lead to depression. Researchers at the Leiden University Medical Center in the Netherlands hypothesize that inflammation, low self-esteem caused by body dissatisfaction and negative endocrine side effects are all linked to depression in the overweight population. Adipose tissue is known to release chemical mediators called interleukins that increase the chance for developing depression. The inflammatory effects of added fat also put the body in a vulnerable state for developing this condition. The stigma and limitations associated with being overweight will further encourage the development depression. Often there is a cyclical relationship between depression and being overweight whereby being overweight means you are at risk of developing depression, and being depressed puts you at a greater risk of being overweight. Luckily, exercise helps combat this trend even before the pounds drop.

▼ **IF YOU ARE PLANNING** to start a family, get your body ready for baby by losing your excess weight before you get pregnant.

7 Liver Disease

Non-alcoholic fatty liver disease (NAFLD) encompasses a range of liver issues from simple fatty liver (steatosis) to non-alcoholic steatosis (NASH) to cirrhosis. These conditions develop when excess fat literally has nowhere else to go and accumulates in the liver. This is often the result of insulin-resistance from type 2 diabetes or metabolic syndrome. NASH has the added insult of liver inflammation, which can lead to cirrhosis and subsequent liver failure. Imagine having the liver of an alcoholic simply by overindulging in processed fare.

8 Pregnancy & Fertility Complications

Weight gain before and during pregnancy puts both mother and baby at risk. Mom is likely to develop insulin resistance, high blood sugar and high blood pressure, which can easily lead to complications such as gestational diabetes, preeclampsia and need for a Cesarean section during delivery. The baby experiences increased risk of developing neural tube defects, being stillborn, undergoing premature delivery and being of large birth weight. Strict dieting to lose excess weight during pregnancy is not recommended because of the chance of depriving the child of nutrients, but losing weight before even trying to get pregnant is ideal and can make the process of conceiving much easier. Sadly one quarter of North American couples are infertile. Infertility amongst overweight couples is common due to ovulatory dysfunction in women and scrotal temperature increases that negatively affect sperm quality in men. Creating a healthy baby starts with your food and activity decisions well before the thought of having a child becomes a reality. It's time to take things very seriously.

9 Gallbladder Disease

Your gallbladder sits behind your liver and concentrates bile to deal aid in fat digestion. When you are overweight you are at major risk of developing one of many gallbladder conditions, such as cholelithiasis (gallstones). Excess fat means bile contains less bile salts and is less able to handle fat digestion. This leads to excess cholesterol production, which then compounds in the gallbladder causing stones and reduced emptying of bile from the gallbladder. This is especially true in

▼ **TREATMENT** for sleep apnea includes wearing a continuous positive airway pressure (CPAP) machine to keep levels of oxygen and carbon dioxide in the blood normal.

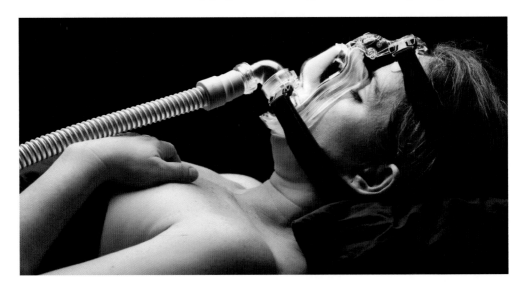

overweight women. This is an uncomfortable condition that puts you at greater risk of developing gallbladder cancer.

10 Sleep Apnea

Sleep apnea is a major problem for overweight individuals, who are at a much higher risk of developing this condition. Added fat around the neck decreases the diameter of the airway, which makes it more difficult to breathe when lying down. This increases the likelihood of snoring and arrested breathing. Chemically, the inflammatory effects of additional fat add to the causative factors of sleep apnea. We spend six to eight hours each day sleeping, and the more comfortable we are, the more soundly we will sleep, the more rested we will be and less heavy we will be.

What To Expect

What should you expect when you begin following the *Eat-Clean Diet Stripped* program? Of course you should expect to lose 10 pounds in 28 days, but what else would you expect? Depending on what you're in the habit of eating, you can expect big changes along with losing the final layer of fat.

The Way You Are Now

Losing the last 10 pounds means different things to different people. Perhaps you are quite lean and already follow a tight diet but you've entered a bikini contest and need a perfectly flat belly. Maybe you have no intention of getting into a two-piece but just want to lose 10 pounds because your clothes have gotten a little tight lately. The *Stripped* program might be a complete transformation of your daily diet or it might be a simple tweak. And as with your goals and eating habits, your starting point is as individual as you are. Each of you will have a unique response to this new exciting eating plan but the common thread will be improved health and excess pounds lost.

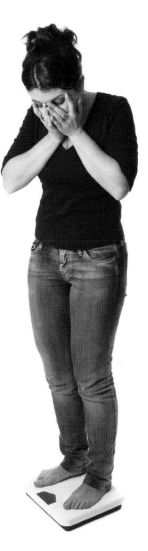

▲ **IF YOU'VE** yo-yo dieted in the past, you know that fad diets and so-called "diet foods" don't work.

> ## "Nothing gives you the high you are going to get from looking and feeling fantastic."

Why are you 10 pounds over the weight you want to be? Do you Eat Clean through the day and binge at night? Do you simply eat whatever you feel like eating? Or is it that you never made the connection between what goes in your mouth and how you look and feel, as I did? Chances are, you've been less than careful with your diet. If you're one of those people who eat a lot of fast food, prepared foods or "diet" versions of your favorite foods, then you can bet you've got lots of chemicals and fake sugars floating around in your bloodstream, all of which end up being stored in your fat cells. You may find that the first few days of this program are not as comfortable as you would hope – you may develop a headache or feel a little sluggish as these toxins leave your body. But once you get past that, look out! You'll be a lion ready to roar! Nothing gives you the high you are going to get from looking and feeling fantastic.

A Belly Full of Nutrition

You may notice immediately upon starting the *Stripped* program that you are eating more food! However the distinction lies in the quality of food you will be eating. Eating more often will stimulate your metabolism. It is scientifically proven that nutritious foods consumed at regular intervals throughout the day keep the metabolism burning at a steady and efficient pace, helping to blast excess fat away. On this program you will eat highly nutritious meals every two-and-a-half to three hours, without fail. Skipping breakfast or any meal is not going to work!

▼ **HIGH-QUALITY** foods include: vegetables, fruits, whole grains, lean proteins, nuts and seeds.

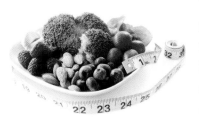

These nutrients flowing through your body on a constant basis, providing your trillions of cells with what they need to thrive, means you should encounter startling positive effects almost immediately. Everywhere in your body, old cells are constantly dying off and new cells are being created. The food you eat dictates what those new cells will be created from. Eating a diet filled with high-quality lean proteins, vitamin- and mineral-rich vegetables and nourishing, fiber-rich starches provides those new cells with optimal building blocks. These nutrients, along with the indispensable water you will be drinking, will also help your body to function at peak performance. The result is nothing short of spectacular.

See the Difference!

When you feed your body Clean, nutrient-rich food and create new cells from superior building materials, you will notice improvements in every area of your body. You may see the difference first in your skin, which will be clear and radiant. Your nails will be stronger and your eyes will be bright. Other changes occur at various levels. Your digestion will improve and you will make daily bowel movements. You will have better-smelling breath and fewer dental caries. When sugar and refined foods are removed from the diet, blood sugar corrects itself to more stable levels of circulating glucose. The skeleton and organs are less prone to mineral loss, common in high-sugar diets. Hormones find a balance once again. You may even find you will have less blood flow during menstruation. Women experiencing menopause generally feel less in the grip of hot flashes, irritability and depressed libido once they begin to Eat Clean. Furthermore, your sleep will be deep and restorative.

Real Hunger

Many of us don't recognize or experience the feeling of hunger. We feed ourselves because food is in front of us, because we're bored or because we're filling an emotional need. Following *The Eat-Clean Diet* means giving your body what it needs, and no more than it needs, at regular intervals. The result is a system that works like a finely made watch. When you wake up in the morning, you'll be ready for a hearty breakfast. Then, around three hours later, you'll be hungry for your next meal, and

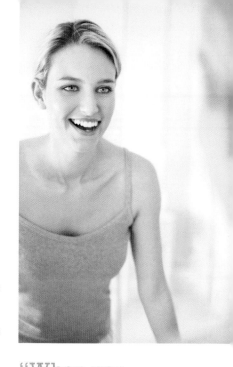

"When you feed your body Clean, nutrient-rich food and create new cells from superior building materials, you will notice improvements in every area of your body."

"Beginning
a weight-loss
diet can often
mean you lose
energy, but not
in this case."

incidentally it will be time for that meal. This will continue until your last meal of the day. We in developed countries are increasingly numb to the experience of hunger because we live in an "obesogenic" society. This new word describes an environment in which many factors combine to predispose us to gaining weight, not the least of which is empty foods.

Understanding the feeling of hunger and knowing what to do about it with the correct tools, including Clean foods, will virtually guarantee your permanent weight-loss success. I'm convinced one of the reasons so many of us are overweight is that we have lost touch with our body's ability to tell us when and how much to eat. Most diets don't help, because they force the dieter to become overly hungry, which is likely to lead to bingeing. Because on this program you have a constant supply of food, after only a week or two you should begin to feel hungry when it's time to eat and satisfied after you have eaten, just as you were designed to.

Energy to Burn

Beginning a weight-loss diet can often mean you lose energy, but not in this case. Because you are providing your body with everything it needs and *not* filling it with sugar, fake sugars, trans fats, chemicals and other negative substances, your body will rejoice and reward you with abundant energy to participate in an active and fulfilled life.

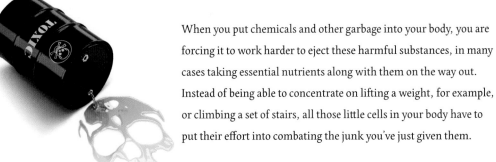

When you put chemicals and other garbage into your body, you are forcing it to work harder to eject these harmful substances, in many cases taking essential nutrients along with them on the way out. Instead of being able to concentrate on lifting a weight, for example, or climbing a set of stairs, all those little cells in your body have to put their effort into combating the junk you've just given them.

Once you stop forcing your trillions of cells to go into constant battle just to survive, they will spend their efforts working for you. Suddenly you'll find you actually feel good when you wake up in the morning. When it's time for your run, or for exercise class, you'll be raring to go. This is especially important when you're trying to lose those last 10 pounds, as you are right now. You'll need to pick it up a little exercise-wise, and getting that extra boost of energy from a squeaky-Clean diet will really help you along.

> "You've got to keep your pipes running clear, and Clean food is the way to do it."

Digestion

You can't feel your best when you're clogged up. Yet some people regularly go days without ... er, going. Talk about a toxic environment! You've got to keep your pipes running clear, and Clean food is the way to do it. This is the case at all times, but especially when you're trying to lose weight. The decrease in food coupled with the lack of quality in most weight-loss diets can mean trouble on the toilet.

▼ **YOU CAN DO** 1,000 sit-ups a day, but the only way to achieve a flat stomach is to Eat Clean.

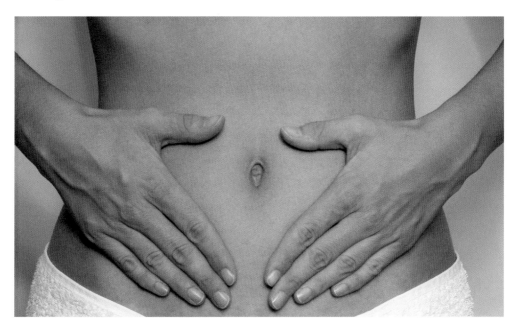

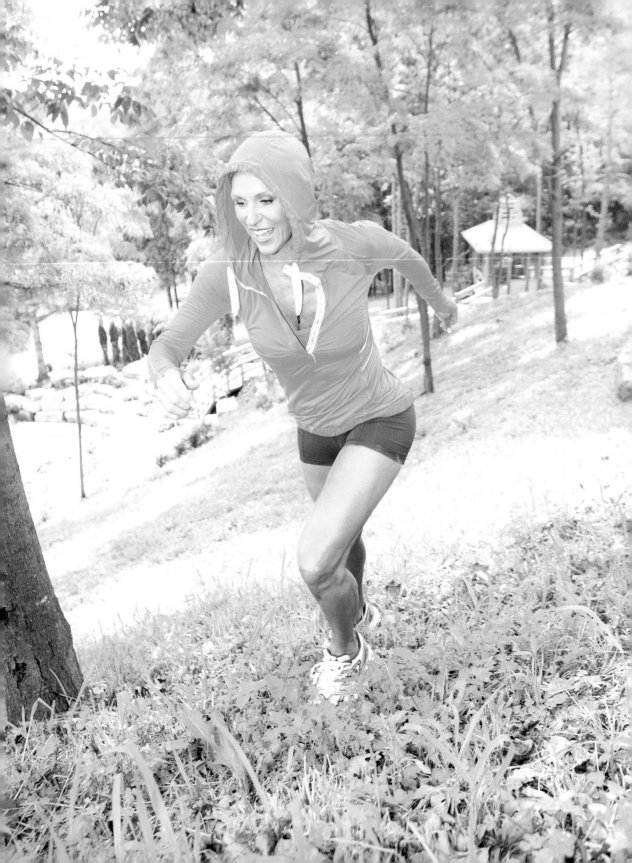

The larger quantity of high-quality foods you'll eat on the *Stripped* plan means your digestive tract should stay in good working order! Our bodies work best when we eat foods packed with nutrition and fiber. The food goes in, breaks down to supply us with what we need, and whatever's left over leaves as quickly as it came. That is a well-functioning body.

Weight Loss

Yes, finally, you will lose weight. In the first few days of your new Eat-Clean Diet lifestyle you will feel lighter without that heavy, greasy food in your belly. Your mid-section will feel slimmer. Then those numbers on the scale will begin moving downward. You may lose a couple of pounds very quickly. Your jeans will stop feeling tight, and then they'll begin to feel loose! You'll have an excuse to buy a new pair. Those tough 10 pounds that have been plaguing you for far too long will be gone, even if you thought you'd never get rid of them.

▼ **GET INSPIRED!** Meet the people who've transformed their bodies and their lives by Eating Clean! Go to eatcleandiet.com/success_stories

No one can make you follow this *Eat-Clean Diet Stripped* program. Ultimately it will be up to you to do what you have to in order to reach your goals. But know that if you do follow this results-oriented program you *will* reach your goals and be slim at last. So over the next 28 days you can expect to feel sensational, with a body that functions better than ever before from head to toe, on the inside and out. You can expect to become in tune with your hunger rhythm and lose the urge to overeat or binge. And as if all that weren't enough, you can expect that unwelcome layer of fat you have – you know the one, it's what makes those rolls when you bend over, hangs overtop your favorite jeans and makes you unwilling to wear a form-fitting dress – that layer of fat will simply disappear. How great is that?!

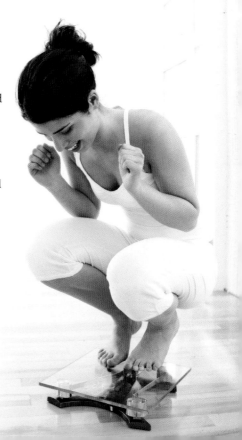

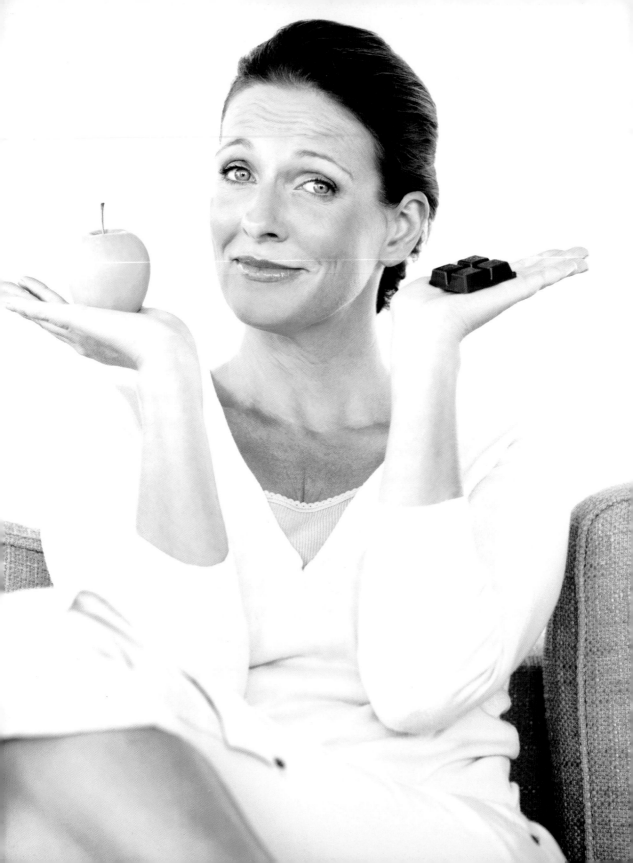

2 | A Nutritional Game Plan

It may surprise you to learn that any change in your eating patterns begins not on your plate, but rather in your head. That billion-celled entity living between your ears (your brain) is entirely responsible for the choices you make regarding the food you eat. You and your brain make a myriad of decisions about how much food to eat, when to eat, what kind of food to consume and so on. This is one of the reasons I send out a caveat to all would-be dieters; be warned!

Your grocery cart, the drive thru, family dinner, potluck, night out on the town and office event – these are all places you could fall into an ocean of trouble. You'll need a nutritional game plan firmly set in your mind before you attempt to tackle your final 10 pounds!

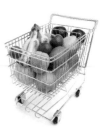

My brain didn't always show up when it came to making decisions about what to eat, particularly at events such as the family-reunion-Grandma's-70th-birthday summer barbecue. My family always does these kinds of multi-purpose events because distance prevents us from gathering more frequently. When the big day arrived an abundance of food appeared as if to ward off the mother of all famines. Like everyone else, I would keep eating until either the weekend was over or the food ran out. It was mindless eating.

Mentally switch on the light bulb over your head. Any attempt at weight loss must begin well before the food appears. In the past I regarded all food as edible and equal, not giving a thought to whether or not it would have ill effect on me. I ate blindly until at one point I weighed 204 pounds. It's all too easy to eat yourself into a situation where you weigh too much, whether 10 or 200 pounds too much.

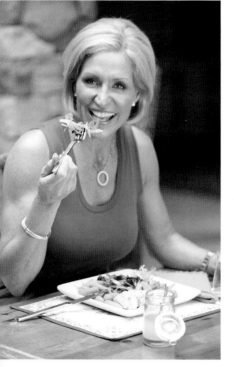

"Mentally switch on the light bulb over your head. Any attempt at weight loss must begin well before the food appears."

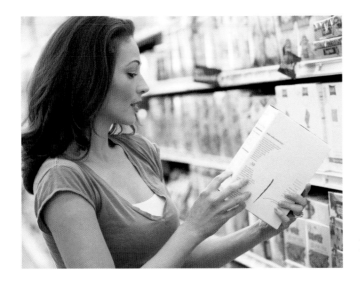

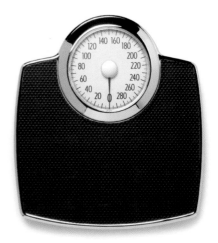

◀ **TO FIND OUT** exactly what you're eating, read the nutrition label on the package. Don't be fooled by flashy marketing claims.

The family barbeque isn't the only place that brings food troubles. The supermarket is just as challenging. People shop when they are in a rush and feel stressed out. Their eyes are half closed and they have no trouble believing every claim on the boxes, packets, bottles and jars that shout, "THIS FOOD IS GOOD FOR YOU!" Let me suggest how idiotic that notion is. Are you going to take your nutritional guidance from a box?

The question is: what *do* you know? I didn't know much because I abandoned myself to the seduction of food marketers. I let myself be guided by what they thought would fool me into parting with my money. Too many of us make food purchases without understanding the repercussions of what that food will do to us, or already has done since we are facing that dreaded 10-pound weight gain at the moment. This is going to change as of now.

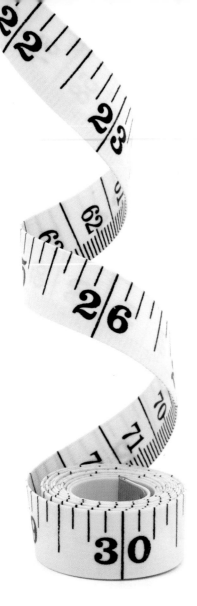

The Plan

A little plan called *The Eat-Clean Diet Stripped* is going to serve as the framework for how you eat from now on, not only to help you shed those last 10 pounds, but afterwards too. I'm excited to introduce *The Eat-Clean Diet* to you if you are a newcomer, because this simple way of eating is transforming the way North Americans eat, one mouthful at a time. This is my plan for you and for all of us. We are sorely in need of overhauling the Standard American Diet (SAD) because it just isn't working for us. We need something new.

For those of you who are not newcomers, welcome back. Since the *Eat-Clean Diet* series began five years ago, well over a million copies have sold and yes, I am proud to say that, but I am prouder to say that the *Eat-Clean Diet* message has affected millions of North Americans positively. These people have not only lost weight, but also improved their health by following the lifestyle. Even if you didn't want to lose a single pound, wouldn't you want to be healthy? Your improved health is the most important thing.

The Eat-Clean Diet makes sense in today's world because it is a sound, lifestyle way of eating based on wholesome foods including lean proteins, whole grains, healthy fats, fresh fruit and vegetables. Over and above consuming such healthy fare, *The Eat-Clean Diet* tells you how much to eat and how frequently. The quantity of food we eat impacts our waistlines as surely as the kinds of foods we eat and how often we eat them. Losing those last 10 requires a little extra diligence, and so in this book I will give you the information you need to accomplish this goal.

But just because I promise a 10-pound weight loss in 28 days doesn't mean this is a fad diet. Far from it! This program is not

"These people have not only lost weight, but improved their health by following the lifestyle."

about counting calories, carbohydrates or fat grams, or weighing your food. And it is most definitely not about starvation. These are substantial claims to make about a diet. In fact, you can call this plan a "Live-It," as many of my readers like to say, because it is a way of living with food that returns you to health and wellness. Fad diets will not do this. *The Eat-Clean Diet Stripped* is based on *The Eat-Clean Diet* but with a tighter approach. I strongly encourage you to consider your nutrition as an essential way of gaining and maintaining your health and weight. "Let your food be your medicine and your medicine be your food," said Hippocrates. And shedding those last 10 pounds will bring about so many positive changes in you and your health!

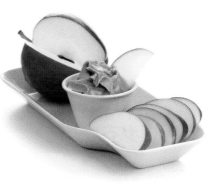

▼ **BY CHOOSING** real food, such as fresh fruits and nut butter, your energy levels will go through the roof!

A Day of Eat-Clean Diet Stripped Eating ✓	A Day of Eating Garbage ✗
MEAL 1: Oatmeal with chopped apple and cinnamon; four scrambled egg whites; coffee and water. ✔	**BREAKFAST:** Coffee with cream and sugar. ✗
MEAL 2: Strawberries and a scant handful of cashews; water. ✔	**MID-MORNING SNACK:** Donut; coffee with cream and sugar. ✗
MEAL 3: Grilled chicken breast sliced overtop raw spinach, black beans, chopped onion and tomato; water. ✔	**LUNCH:** Ham and cheese sandwich on white bread with mayo; apple; small packet of chips; regular soft drink. ✗
MEAL 4: One hardboiled egg; half a banana; water. ✔	**MID-AFTERNOON SNACK:** Chocolate bar; regular soft drink. ✗
MEAL 5: Baked salmon; half a baked sweet potato; roasted Brussels sprouts; water. ✔	**DINNER:** Three slices of pizza; garlic bread; Caesar salad; beer. ✗
MEAL 6 (if hungry): One sliced apple spread with almond butter; water. ✔	**AFTER-DINNER SNACK:** Pretzels from the bag; regular soft drink. ✗

ONE OF THE BEST THINGS ABOUT *THE EAT-CLEAN DIET* LIFESTYLE is that it's flexible. If you suffer from food allergies, intolerances or simply do not like certain foods, plan a menu around your dietary issues by following the *Eat-Clean Diet* Principles (page 52) and consuming foods that don't cause you any trouble or discomfort.

The following foods account for 90 percent of food allergic reactions, according to the U.S. Food and Drug Administration:

❶ Milk

❷ Eggs

❸ Fish
(bass, flounder, cod)

❹ Crustacean shellfish
(crab, lobster, shrimp)

❺ Tree nuts (almonds, walnuts, pecans)

❻ Peanuts

❼ Wheat

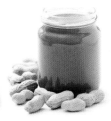

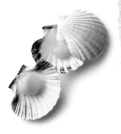

If You Can't Eat...	Try...
Milk	Rice, soy, almond or oat milk
Eggs	Tofu 1 Tbsp ground flax + 3 Tbsp water (in baking)
Fish	Alternative protein (chicken, turkey, bison, beans, tofu, etc.)
Shellfish	Alternative protein (lean beef, lean pork, edamame, seitan, protein powder, etc.)
Tree nuts	Sunflower, pumpkin and sesame seeds
Peanuts/peanut butter	Soy nuts/butter, sunflower seeds/butter
Wheat	Rice, potato, sorghum or bean flours Tapioca or Potato starch Gluten-free breads and products
Soybeans	Meat proteins, beans (red, black, kidney, etc.) and lentils, nuts and nut butters

Many readers write to me asking whether they must consume foods they do not like in order to meet their goals. The answer is definitely not! Just because I eat oatmeal and egg whites every morning for breakfast does not mean you have to as well. You can eat anything you like, so long as you are following the *Eat-Clean Diet* Principles (for an at-a-glance list of the Principles, see page 67).

Here are some common foods I am asked about and their appropriate substitutions:

If You Dislike...	Try...
Eggs	Any other protein, including chicken, beans, protein powder, etc.
Oatmeal	Any other starchy complex carbohydrate including bananas, whole grain toast, brown rice, etc.
Sweet potatoes	White potatoes, winter squash
Fish	Any other protein including pork tenderloin, edamame, bison, protein powder, etc.

"You can eat anything you like, so long as you are following the *Eat-Clean Diet* Principles."

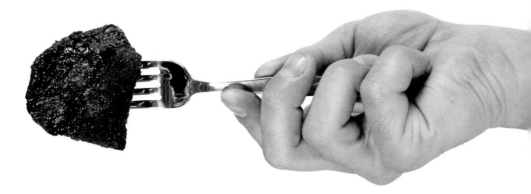

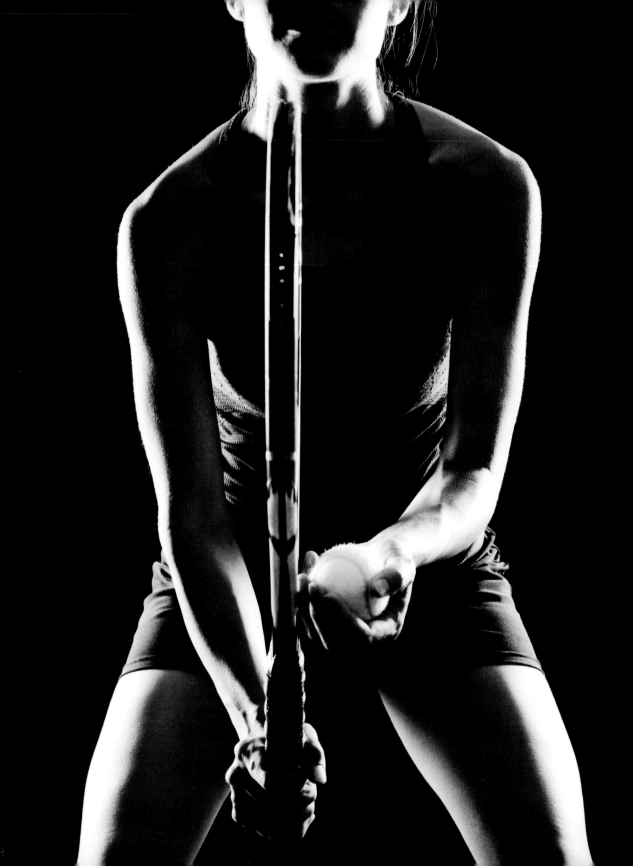

3 | Getting Your Game Face On

A nutritional game plan will get you off on the best start possible. Be prepared – get your game face on before every meal, ready to stare down your dinner plate. Tennis pro Venus Williams would never consider taking on an opponent unless she understood her game strategy intimately. She would do her research, find out all she could about her challenger, study the plays, the previous wins and losses, and then she would plan her approach. She would also get her body in the best physical condition possible. All successful people prepare themselves for upcoming tasks.

> **"Studies show having a plan accounts for 75 percent of your success. The rest is just execution."**

Taking a note from Venus's highly decorated career, we too should have a well-defined attack planned out as we undertake the physical challenge we have set for ourselves – to shed those last 10 pounds. A nutritional game plan is your tennis ace, your birdie or your home run. Without it you are much more likely to fail. Studies show having a plan accounts for 75 percent of your success. The rest is just execution.

Telling Your Story

Part of getting your game face on involves writing down your goals. The simple act of writing down your intention to lose weight automatically makes you 50 percent more likely to succeed at the task you have set for yourself. So write this down on a piece of paper, in a journal or somewhere you can see it every day:

I am going to lose 10 pounds in 28 days!
I'll do it by following the Eat-Clean Diet Stripped *program!*

Already you are 50 percent more likely to succeed! Good for you! I like to record things like this in a journal because I believe the front and back covers give me some privacy, while the pages in between give me the freedom to write anything and everything. The journal I use has to have a place for me to record my goals, my successes, my errors and plateaus, my training and also my eating. There are numerous computer programs wherein you can log this information, but I am a little old fashioned and enjoy the feel of paper and pencil when I scribble down these details. Your daily journal pages will add up and ultimately you'll have your own story, an entire book describing your journey of losing 10 pounds. If the computer works for you or if you prefer a phone application then go ahead and use it – just get it down.

At last count I had over 20 journals filled with my training and eating information, details about when I might have competed, whether I was ill or any other possibly relevant tidbits. These books are my record of what I am capable of with regard to training and eating. I often flip through the pages of earlier journals to remind myself of how far I have come, and to note any changes or trends.

Your book could be a best seller. It is filled with riveting stuff! Your story is fantastic. It's empowering. There is a wonderful beginning where your struggle is laid out: "I need to lose 10 pounds fast!" Next you need to clarify why you are doing this. An example might be, "I have to lose this weight because I am getting married in 28 days and I want to look amazing!" Mine would read, "I need to lose 10 pounds in 28 days because I am competing in the Miss Bikini America contest. I want to come in tight and I don't want to embarrass myself among the other competitors."

Along the way, factors will add to or subtract from your level of success. Write these down too. You may write something such as, "I have the flu so I can't train." My story would read something like, "I have to travel for business and there's no gym at the hotel. Had to make do with bodyweight exercises." Whatever your story is, write it down. Record your daily meals including what you ate, what time you ate it and how you felt at that time.

I also pencil down how I felt during my workouts. Sometimes I write things like, "I feel strong in the legs today" or "I totally trashed my abs." I usually scribble in big letters my great accomplishments such as, "I ran 10 very hilly kilometers today without stopping!" I like those days.

"If you want to obliterate those fatty 10 pounds you've got to take journaling seriously."

Other characters may show up in your story. I often train with different people and I make that part of my tale: "Today I trained with Elaine Goodlad. She kicked my butt." Sometimes I run with my daughter so I note that too: "I ran 10 kilometers with Kiersten today and she really challenged me."

I need to record details like this because they help me stay focused and motivated, which encourages me to stick with my plan and succeed. My notes serve as a reminder of why I'm doing what I'm doing. If you forget why you're waking up an hour early to run or hitting the gym after work, go back to the beginning of your journal and reread that first line that states your goal:

I am going to lose 10 pounds in 28 days!

Reread this statement as many times as you need to! If you want to obliterate those fatty 10 pounds you've got to take journaling seriously. The final 10 are a different breed than the previous 100, 50 or 20 pounds. They are stubborn, difficult and finicky, and you have to be more determined to get rid of them than they are to stay put. Be warned!

Be In Position

Someone I admire very much, Robin Roberts, co-anchor on *Good Morning America*, explains in her recent best-selling book *From the Heart: Eight Rules to Live By*, that being in the correct position for success is one of her most important rules. She writes, "I'm a big believer that you have to put yourself in position for good things to happen to you. You can dream, hope and pray all you want but if you're not ready when the opportunity calls, it will pass you by." This relates to my point about getting your game face on.

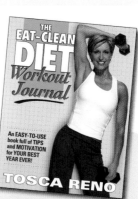

▶ **FOOD JOURNALING** helps you stay aware of what you're eating so you can stay on plan.

WEEKLY FOOD TRACKER

DATE Monday, May 2

MORNING START	Oatmeal with berries, bee pollen, flaxseed and wheat germ; egg whites; water and coffee.
MIDMORNING MUNCH	Nonfat plain yogurt with strawberries; water.
LUNCHTIME REFUEL	Whole grain pasta with chopped fresh tomatoes; grilled chicken; water.

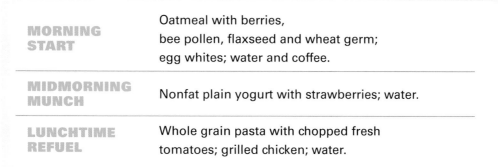

▶ **TRAINING JOURNALS** are an invaluable tool for tracking progress and breaking through plateaus.

YOUR TRAINING JOURNAL

TRAINING Monday, May 2

BODY PART	EXERCISE		SET 1	SET 2	SET 3
Chest	Bench Press	WEIGHT	60 lbs	85 lbs	85 lbs
		REPS	8	8	8
Upper Back	Bent-Over Rows	WEIGHT	50 lbs	70 lbs	70 lbs
		REPS	10	10	10
Thighs	Squats	WEIGHT	60 lbs	110 lbs	120 lbs
		REPS	10	10	10

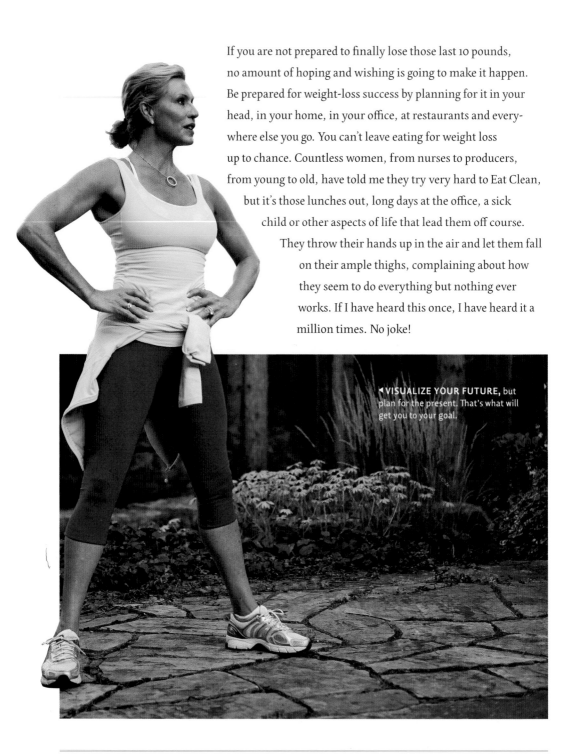

If you are not prepared to finally lose those last 10 pounds, no amount of hoping and wishing is going to make it happen. Be prepared for weight-loss success by planning for it in your head, in your home, in your office, at restaurants and everywhere else you go. You can't leave eating for weight loss up to chance. Countless women, from nurses to producers, from young to old, have told me they try very hard to Eat Clean, but it's those lunches out, long days at the office, a sick child or other aspects of life that lead them off course. They throw their hands up in the air and let them fall on their ample thighs, complaining about how they seem to do everything but nothing ever works. If I have heard this once, I have heard it a million times. No joke!

◄ **VISUALIZE YOUR FUTURE,** but plan for the present. That's what will get you to your goal. ►

Of course it doesn't work. How could it possibly? You can't make a plan to lose 10 pounds and then let loose at the buffet counter because it's a co-worker's birthday lunch. If you want to be successful at dropping excess pounds then you must employ what every other successful person has employed: optimization. This means you attack a problem from every angle, doing everything possible to come up with a solution. Even more important, you try to think of the solutions before the problems arise. This is what *The Eat-Clean Diet Stripped* is all about.

I was recently at the offices of a huge national television show. Several of the staff approached me, wanting to know how they could lose a few pounds. I explained about how following this lifestyle would mean eating more food and eating more frequently. They looked at me like they didn't really grasp what I was trying to explain. Instead of repeating myself, I invited them to come and have a look at my cooler bag, which I had packed that morning, so I would have something nutritious and Clean to reach for during my busy day. Together those women and I pulled out each item from the cooler. Showing them my daily eats helped them understand how easy it is to position yourself for weight-loss success by optimizing your efforts. (To see what I put in my cooler, visit: **www.eatcleandiet.com/ toscascooler**.) Leaving your eating to chance displaces your efforts and puts you square in the path of foods that won't help you drop a single pound.

Packing a cooler positions you successfully for answering hunger pangs during your busy workday. It is one of the Eat-Clean Diet Principles – which you will learn all about in the next chapter – that is a must.

"If you do not put yourself in the position of being prepared you will not reach your goal."

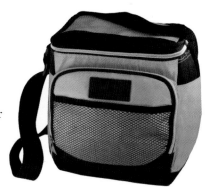

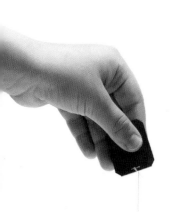

> "There is an enormous emotional element both to eating and to losing weight."

If you do not put yourself in the position of being prepared you will not reach your goal. You will allow prevailing circumstances to decide what you are going to eat. Without readiness and preparedness there is no successful result. You might as well eat a big hunk of chocolate cake and continue to gain weight!

A Strategy For Weight-Loss Success

You and I know that dropping those pounds for good is really about having a solid strategy. There is an enormous emotional element both to eating and to losing weight. At a recent seminar I shared my story of how I had become so terribly overweight. I had derived a tremendous amount of comfort from eating peanut butter, a trigger food. "I just couldn't figure out how to put the lid on the jar," I shared. The entire room burst into laughter. Apparently many of us have the same problem!

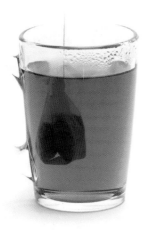

A good strategy for me was to stop eating peanut butter and stop buying it altogether. We each have at least one trigger food (and you may have many). Whatever yours is, you must first identify it as a trigger food. If you can't stop eating it once you start, then eliminate it from your diet for the time being. It is best to have it out of sight and way out of mind for a while, until you reach your goal of losing 10 pounds.

You may have to reprogram your brain to help you avoid your trigger foods. Rewire your thinking. Here is how I do it: When I feel the urge to indulge in cheese (another trigger food), I remind myself of my goal to lose and why I want to do it. "Oh yes! I will be onstage in a bikini in a few weeks. Better not eat that cheese." Then I make myself a cup of tea, which keeps my hands busy, and I leave the kitchen. I hope the cheese demons are gone by the time I have finished my tea – they usually are.

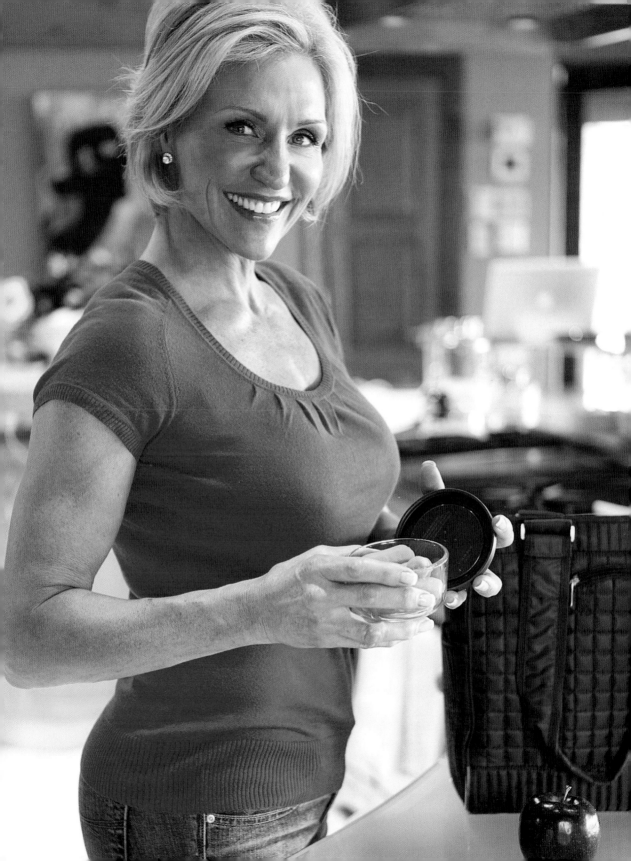

BRINGING YOUR LUNCH TO WORK is of the utmost importance if you are going to reach your *Stripped* weight-loss goals. From experience, I know there aren't many restaurants offering the Clean eats I need to fuel my body regularly. That's why I bring my meals with me everywhere I go!

Brown bagging my lunch ensures that I stay on track with my diet, and I save money along the way – can't beat that! The best part about always having Clean food on hand is that it prevents you from grabbing food in a hurry, food that may not keep you on your plan of shedding those last 10 pounds.

Here are some practical strategies to help you Eat Clean, get *Stripped* lean and still make it to work on time without starving yourself.

Bon appétit!

① Pack your lunch in a cooler bag.

A cooler bag doesn't just carry your meals, it also prevents food spoilage by keeping your food cool and free from bacteria. In addition to my lunch, I also add a frozen ice pack to my cooler bag to ensure my meals stay cold and fresh for many hours. You can find cooler bags at most major retailers in all sizes, colors and price ranges. Buy several back-up ice packs – for some reason they go missing frequently.

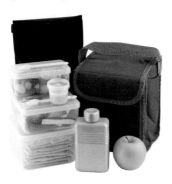

② You can never have too many containers.

I have a mountain of containers – in all shapes and sizes – in my cupboards. I try to have enough to pack planned leftovers for everyone's lunches at night without scrambling to wash the ones I used that day. Then I throw the dirty containers in the dishwasher and let that magic machine do its work! Currently I have a preference for glass containers with see-through lids. You may think glass is dangerous, but if you pack your cooler correctly your glass container will be safe and you will benefit from not being exposed to BPAs present in most plastic containers.

③ Keep your staples at the office.

My office and the company fridge hold a treasure chest of my Clean goods! I keep oatmeal, soymilk, almonds, dried fruit, balsamic vinegar, nut butter and a number of other Eat-Clean essentials at work at all times. This way I don't have to lug too many items to work each day and I have Clean staples to rely on if I'm short on food and time. What a relief it is to know I always have access to Clean foods that will keep me nourished and on track for shedding a few pounds.

④ Freeze food.

Make large batches of soup, stews and chili, and freeze them in individual containers. When you're short on time, you can throw one in your bag and your lunch will be thawed by the time you're ready for it. This is an invaluable way to save money and save time in the kitchen.

⑤ Prevent soggy lunches.

Soggy lunches are unappealing and unappetizing on many different levels. I keep ingredients such as tomatoes, salad dressing and balsamic vinegar in small containers until I'm ready to add them to my lunch. My salads stay crisp and my hummus doesn't turn my brown rice wraps into goo by the time I'm ready to eat them. Any foods with a high water or fat content should be wrapped individually.

⑥ Clean your cooler or lunch bag often.

Wipe your cooler bag with soap and warm water at least once a week to clean out any food scraps that may be left behind. This will remove germs from the bag and prevent it from being odorous! I have on occasion discovered my daughter's cooler that has been left under a pile of school papers in her room for several days – most unpleasant!

⑦ Make lunch a culinary experience.

I create the experience of a fine dining restaurant wherever I go. I keep a plate, cutlery and placemats in my office and use them every day. I set a place for myself in my lunchroom and arrange my food nicely on my plate. I savor my food, enjoying the lunch I have packed for myself. I am always satisfied at the end of the meal and I return to my desk with a clear head ready to work for the afternoon!

Attaching Emotion To Your Efforts

In this plan to shed weight there is a need for emotion, but it must be attached to your goals. Motivational speaker Zig Ziglar has declared that when you attach emotion to your efforts, you triple your chances for success. Find your emotional juggernaut. The reason you want to lose weight should be substantial enough to carry you through your efforts.

My original transformation was inspired for two reasons – one, I'd seen myself in a photograph where my children looked slim and vital with their whole lives ahead of them. I looked like I was heading in the opposite direction. I had also watched my father struggle with heart disease and knowing this was a family health risk, I didn't look back. I embraced the healthy Eat-Clean Diet lifestyle immediately. The last 10 pounds may not be so urgent, but you have to find your own emotional connection to that weight loss.

A Word About Cravings

I've never met anyone who hasn't experienced a craving at some point, otherwise known as an intense longing for a particular type of food. Cravings are a bit unpredictable, but in my mind there are two very different kinds: cravings that urge you to eat certain foods rich in a particular nutrient and cravings that relate to boredom, your emotions and tiredness.

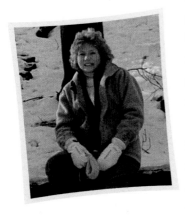

▲ **PHOTOGRAPHS** were not my friend at age 39 (as seen above). Today I love having my photo taken.

Some people experience cravings because their diet is lacking in nutrients. The food they eat is deficient in essential vitamins and minerals. Millions of North Americans struggle with this. A whopping 67 percent of us are overweight or obese and yet we are also starving. How can this be? It scrambles my brains to think about this but it is the truth. When we eat foods lacking in nutritional quality (I like to call these "anti" foods), we are never truly satisfied or satiated. Our bodies sense this. After we consume "anti" foods such as processed white sugar and flour products, the stomach sphincter does not close. It is as if the stomach is still waiting for the arrival of nutrition because it has not recognized the junk you just ate as quality goods. You feel as if you're still hungry even though you're crammed full.

When you feed your body nutritious foods, such as a grilled chicken breast alongside two cups of steamed mixed vegetables and half a cup of brown rice, you feel satiated. Your stomach has received the mother lode and is happily working its way through this goodness. Your stomach needs three hours to process Clean eats so the sphincter closes and you feel full. There is no need to stuff any more food down there – the cravings are gone.

Plenty of of women crave chocolate before or during their menstrual cycle. Here the body is "telling" you that it needs calcium and magnesium. If you must eat chocolate then do as I do and eat dark chocolate that is 75 percent or more in cocoa mass. This is the most nutritious kind of chocolate and it is not wrong to call it "food." Just keep in mind that chocolate, no matter how many healthful ingredients, is still high in fats and at least a little sugar, so you can't eat it with abandon or you will have to forget about losing those last 10 pounds.

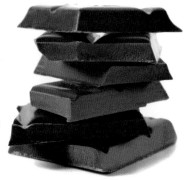

Another common craving is foods with a cold, creamy texture. The food that immediately comes to my mind is ice cream, but that got me squeezing into a size 16 pair of pants so I won't go there again! Instead I reach for plain low-fat yogurt sweetened with unsweetened applesauce or fresh fruit. It does the trick!

"Eat dark chocolate that is 75 percent or more in cocoa mass."

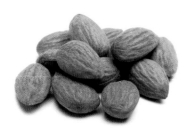

When the need for something to crunch hits I reach for raw, unsalted nuts, particularly almonds and walnuts, to satisfy the need – however, there is a strong caveat here. There is a tremendous tendency to eat nuts mindlessly because they are good for you – this is bad news! Measure out a quarter-cup of nuts and put the rest away, otherwise you will eat the whole bag and be up 10 pounds instead of heading in the opposite direction. I have helped numerous people lose weight simply by identifying nuts as the culprit and eliminating them from daily eating, at least until an ideal weight has been reached.

In the 10 years I've been living the Eat-Clean Diet lifestyle, I have noticed another kind of craving – the kind relating to boredom and tiredness. When I am exhausted (this happens often) or bored (this rarely happens) I find myself reaching for food. Most people I have talked to verify that this happens to them too. Some of us like crunchy things and others want creamy things. This is definitely the time to recognize you are either tired or bored or both and get yourself either busy or to bed, and fast. Otherwise, mayhem will break out in your kitchen and you won't be able to stop yourself from the munchie attack about to unfold.

Are You In the Game?

It's your turn now. Pick up a pen and grab your journal. Jot down your goals for weight loss right now. Ten pounds gone in 28 days is achievable. It is within reach. Come on, you can do it. Four weeks is nothing! Are you in the game? And remember this little piece of wisdom from Zig Ziglar: *"Unless you have definite, precise, clearly set goals you are not going to realize the maximum potential that lies within you."*

"Unless you have definite, precise, clearly set goals you are not going to realize the maximum potential that lies within you."

How to Conquer Cravings

CRAVINGS ARE LARGELY PREVENTABLE and if they do strike, they can be overcome. If you suffer from occasional (or constant!) food cravings, the following guide will help you kick those cravings to the curb.

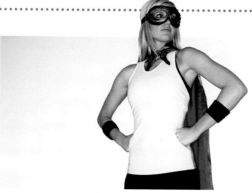

① Determine the source of your craving and get to the root of it.

Have you eaten balanced meals including one or two servings of starchy complex carbohydrates that day? If you aren't feeling satisfied by your meals, it might cause you to crave other foods.

Are you simply thirsty? It's common to mistake thirst for hunger. Try quenching your craving with a tall glass of water or steaming mug of herbal tea.

Do you always crave chocolate at that time of the month? Sometimes it's best to listen to your body and give it what it wants, so long as you practice portion control and don't make it an everyday (or even every week) habit.

② Distract yourself.

Close the kitchen and try any of the following activities:

- Go for a walk
- Talk to a friend on the phone
- Paint your nails (you can't eat while your nails are wet!)
- Take a bath
- Garden
- Hit the gym

Visit The Kitchen Table at www.eatcleandiet.com. Vent about your craving by posting a blog entry and look at other members' stories and photos for motivation.

③ Satisfy your craving in a Clean way.*

Craving sweets? Have fresh berries or a handful of unsweetened dried fruits.

Craving salt? Try unbuttered, air-popped popcorn, homemade baked pita chips and salsa, or a handful of nuts.

*You can turn practically any meal into a Clean one. If your favorite meal is steak and mashed potatoes, make it Clean by using a lean cut of meat and potatoes made with unsweetened almond milk or stock instead of butter. If you crave pizza (during your weight-maintenance plan), load up a whole grain pita with tomatoes, fresh veggies, lean meats and a small amount of nonfat cheese. Making your old favorites Clean will satisfy your cravings without derailing your progress.

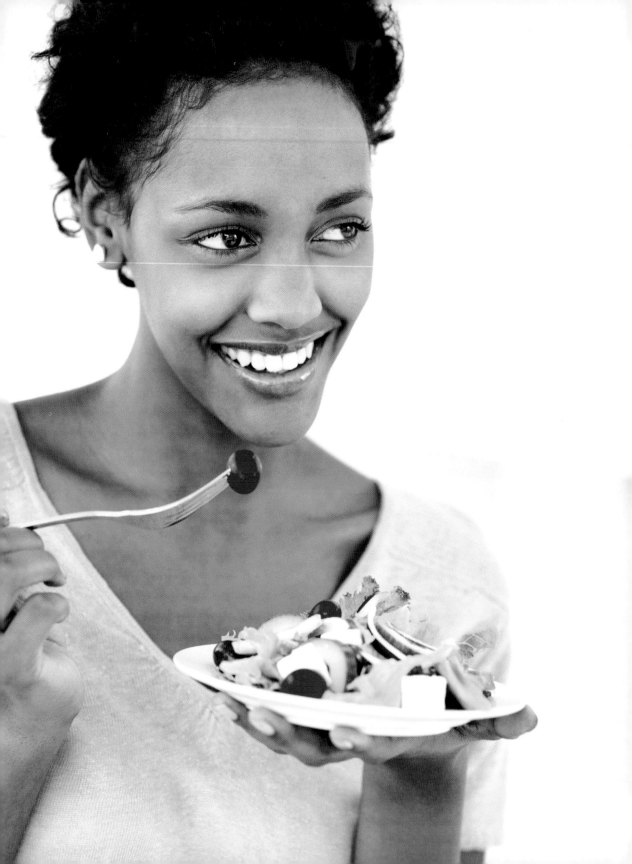

4 | The Eat-Clean Diet Principles

You now know that how you look and feel is primarily the result of what and how often you eat. Your workouts and genetics are each only 10 percent responsible for the body you desire. The bulk of it – 80 percent – is a result of the food you put into your mouth.

> "If you simply want to lose that last lingering bit of weight that's been hanging on for dear life no matter what you do, bookmark this chapter."

The Eat-Clean Diet Principles chapter is your guidebook. Think of the following 10 Principles as rules to live by. If you already own one of my *Eat-Clean Diet* books such as *The Eat-Clean Diet, Expanded Edition* or *The Eat-Clean Diet Recharged!*, I advise you to make note of the changes in this chapter. The Principles in *Stripped* have been designed for you specifically, the person with 10 pounds or less to lose.

Your *Eat-Clean Diet Stripped* eating plan is strict, but it promises results. These Principles are designed to get you where you want to be. If you want to look good for a vacation or special event, this plan is for you. If you're stuck in a weight-loss plateau, this plan will help you get past it. If you simply want to lose that last lingering bit of weight that's been hanging on for dear life no matter what you do, bookmark this chapter.

I could simply give you menu plans and tell you to follow them, but I want you to understand *how* Eating Clean works and *why* it's the best plan to help you reach not only your best weight, but also your best health.

1 Eat more! Eat six small meals each day, spaced at two-and-a-half to three-hour intervals.

Most people are under the impression that they need to starve themselves to lose weight. They equate eating less food with weighing less. Believe me when I tell you that this is a dieting **myth**! When you deprive yourself of nutrition, your body assumes that food is scarce and hangs onto everything you feed it with ferocity, making it difficult to lose weight. This diet mentality also wreaks havoc on your metabolism, slowing it down and confusing your body. Long-term weight loss is never the result!

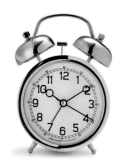

Thankfully there is a way to regulate your metabolism and turn your body into a calorie-burning, fat-blasting machine. How? By eating more food more often. Instead of eating three large meals, you will eat five to six smaller meals each day, spaced out every two-and-a-half to three hours. This frequency causes your metabolism to be constantly stimulated and prevents you from getting too hungry between meals. It may seem counter-intuitive to eat more but this is how I have managed to become the house-wife who lost weight and kept it off for 11 years and counting.

Now that you are eating more often, you will have to make your portions smaller. The idea is to eat the right kinds of foods often enough in the proper amounts to never experience hunger pangs. Every meal is an event that fuels your metabolism and pushes you forward on the path to your best health. Think of each meal also as an opportunity. Yes, an opportunity to do something good for yourself both health- and weight-wise.

2 Eat breakfast every day, within an hour of rising.

"Breakfast is the most important meal of the day" may be a cli-ché, but it's absolutely true! So many people skip breakfast in an attempt to reduce their daily calorie intake, but eating breakfast actually helps you lose weight. The National Weight Control Registry found that those who shed 30 pounds of weight or more did so with the help of eating breakfast. It's also been proven that early eaters consume less saturated fat and cholesterol over the course of the day than someone who skips breakfast.

I eat breakfast because it starts up all of my engines. As soon as you take your first bite of a healthy breakfast, your body awakens and your metabolism starts making use of the energy it gets

WHAT DOES A TYPICAL DAY OF EATING LOOK LIKE?

7:00 AM	Meal #1 or Breakfast
10:00 AM	Meal #2 or Mid-morning
1:00 PM	Meal #3 or Lunch
4:00 PM	Meal #4 or Mid-afternoon
7:00 PM	Meal #5 or Dinner
10:00 PM	Meal #6 or Evening*

MAKE IT WORK FOR YOU: Adjust your schedule to suit your waking, working and eating time.

HUNGRY? You may want to eat every two-and-a-half hours, depending on how active you are during the day.

*Please note that Meal #6 is optional. You should eat this meal only if you are truly, physically hungry. If you are simply bored, make a cup of herbal tea and step out of the kitchen!

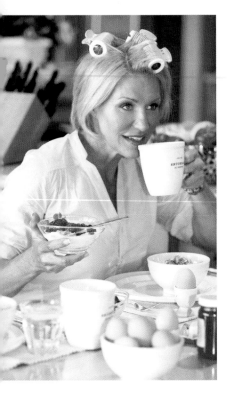

from food. Your brain function is also improved by this morning meal. According to the American Dietetic Association, "Eating breakfast encourages increased concentration and problem-solving skills throughout the day." By skipping breakfast, you are missing out on essential nutrients.

Nobody in my house escapes without an Eat-Clean breakfast. I can't even turn on my computer without my necessary morning start: oatmeal with fresh berries, flaxseed, wheat germ and bee pollen, with a side of scrambled or boiled egg whites. Oatmeal is full of soluble and insoluble plant fibers that slowly break down in your digestive system, giving you a prolonged feeling of fullness that will last until your next meal. Breakfast is non-negotiable with me!

Many people ask me if they should eat something before their early-morning workout. The answer is yes! During the night your blood sugar lowers and your glycogen stores deplete, which translates into a weaker workout. To make the most of your workout, eat before you go, and eat your second mini meal (meal #2 or mid-morning) when you return.

3 Make your last meal three hours before bed.

Can you feel when you are hungry? What does it feel like? Learn to recognize the true signs of hunger in your body: a growling stomach, irritability and the inability to concentrate. Make your best effort to distinguish between real physical hunger and emotional hunger, which is usually the result of boredom, depression, anxiety or a social situation such as a party. You also may feel hungry when you are in fact thirsty. The next time you are hungry after dinner, try drinking a tall glass of water first and see how you feel. Decide afterwards if you are truly hungry or not. You might be surprised to discover how often you mistake thirst for hunger.

My rule for your evening or sixth meal is this: If you are physically hungry, eat! I usually eat my last meal of the day between 9:00 PM and 10:00 PM. As an active woman, I need nutrients and let's face it – I'm hungry! But I don't go overboard. My evening meals are typically smaller and lighter than the rest of my daily eats. For example, I might eat an apple with a handful of raw, unsalted nuts or scrambled egg whites with slices of tomato. But it stops there! I don't reach for ice cream or potato chips because I think I deserve it. No way!

Dinner is usually the biggest meal of the day for North American families, but it doesn't make sense to fill yourself up with energy you won't burn off after dinner. More of your daily nutrition should be consumed at the beginning of the day when you are more likely to be busy and have a better chance at burning the energy away. Judge for yourself if you are going to need this last meal of the day to get you through the night.

"Make your best effort to distinguish between real physical hunger and emotional hunger."

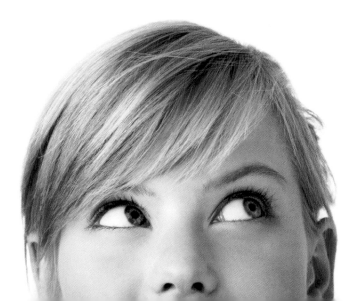

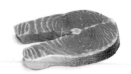

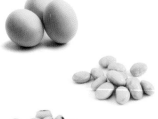

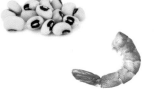

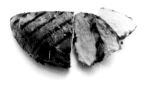

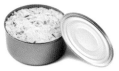

4 Eat a combination of lean protein and complex carbohydrates at each meal.

The frequency of your meals is important, but nothing compares to your food choices. When you choose high-grade foods as your fuel of preference, instead of high-fat, sugar-laden "anti" foods, you are rewarded by increased energy levels and a sense that you are doing right by your body.

Nutrient-dense foods make all the difference. By combining lean protein and complex carbohydrates at each meal, you slow down the carb-to-fat conversion in your body, keeping you satiated between meals.

PROTEIN

Protein is often overlooked in weight-loss regimens. There could be no bigger mistake. Protein is *the* lean bodybuilding food. Strive to eat five to six servings of protein each day, one with each of your mini meals. Protein is primarily found in meat, poultry, fish and eggs but is also found in dairy and to some degree in vegetable and grain sources.

▲ **BODYBUILDERS** and fitness models eat protein at every one of their five or six daily meals.

ALLOWABLE PROTEIN SOURCES INCLUDE:

Egg whites, lean turkey, chicken and pork, beans and legumes (in moderation), lean fish, shrimp, clams, mussels, bison and other game meats, hummus (also a healthy fat), quinoa, spirulina, sea vegetables, protein powder, tofu and tempeh.

COMPLEX CARBOHYDRATES

There are two types of carbohydrates: simple and complex. Simple carbohydrates, such as white flour and sugar, are also known as sugars. They break down easily and tend to send blood-sugar levels out of control. Avoid simple carbs except fruit – fruit contains fiber, which slows its digestion; fruit also contains vital nutrients and minerals.

Complex carbohydrates are high in fiber and improve digestion. They provide you with energy, keep you satisfied between meals and stabilize blood-sugar levels. Consider stabilized blood-sugar levels as the key to keeping hunger in check. Vegetables, fruits and whole grains are all complex carbs.

To break it down even further, there are two types of complex carbohydrates: starchy and high-water. In your *Stripped* menu plan, you will eat two servings of starchy complex carbs and five to six servings of high-water complex carbs each day.

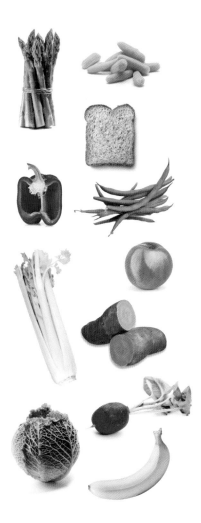

STARCHY COMPLEX CARBOHYDRATES INCLUDE:
Sweet potatoes, potatoes, radishes, beans and legumes (also a protein), oats, brown rice, bananas, carrots, parsnips, bulgar wheat, teff and farro.

COMPLEX CARBS FROM FRUITS AND VEGETABLES:
Apples, plums, berries, pears, tomatoes, cucumber, broccoli, asparagus, beets, leeks, dark leafy greens, Brussels sprouts, green beans, onions, sprouts, celery, watermelon, cherries, zucchini, fennel, oranges, limes, lemons and garlic.

▲ COMPLEX CARBS provide your body with the energy you need to live an active life.

5 Eat sufficient healthy fats every day.

Fat is bad, right? The answer is: not always. Excess fat is not desirable but enough fat to make you and I healthy human beings is. Fat is part of our physical makeup and we need fats – healthy ones – in our diet to function properly. The brain particularly depends on healthy fats to perform properly.

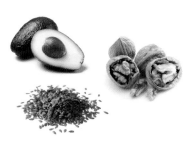

▲ HEALTHY FATS from avocados, nuts and seeds help your body process and burn fat.

FATS — THE BAD GUYS

→ Trans fats

→ Saturated fats – an excess of saturated fats from animal products

→ Man-made fats such as margarine

In your *Stripped* menu plan you should eat one or two servings of healthy fats each day. Allowable sources include: nuts and nut butters, and seeds including flaxseed.

Consuming only "low-fat" or "fat free" products does not solve anyone's fat problem. That diet trend has thankfully come and gone. You need fats to stay slim, but you need the right kind of fats, specifically the fatty acids known as omega-3 and omega-6. These hard-working fats keep cells in a fat-burning or thermogenic state, which is exactly what you want to help you blast off those last 10 pounds.

ALLOWABLE HEALTHY FATS INCLUDE:
Flaxseed, nuts such as almonds and walnuts, pumpkin seeds (in moderation), nut butters, hummus (also a protein), avocados, oils (flaxseed, sesame, coconut, olive, hazelnut, walnut and fish).

6 Drink two to three liters of water each day.

Water should be the drink you reach for before all else. It is the very basis of life and is critical to your Eat-Clean game plan. Both losing and maintaining weight depend on adequate hydration. I've made it easy for you by programming water into each of your daily meals.

Water is second only to oxygen in the level of importance it has to the body. Roughly 75 percent of your body is water, the bulk of which is stored in the largest organ, your skin. Water regulates your body temperature, keeps joints mobile and maintains tissue health. When you become dehydrated the trillions of cells housed in your body are threatened with breakdown and damage in the face of insufficient water. You need water to survive.

Weight loss cannot occur without water. Your metabolic rate increases by as much as 30 percent when you drink cold water because your body must work harder to bring the temperature of

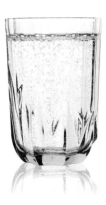

▲ **DRINK A GLASS** of water during each of your five to six daily mini meals. You'll stay full and hydrated.

the water up to that of your body. Get used to reaching for water as your beverage of choice.

Use water to prevent thirst, instead of making the mistake of reaching for it after you are already thirsty – then it is too late. The headache has already kicked in. You feel sluggish, even irritable. When I am thirsty I often mistake the feeling for being hungry and feel the urge to nibble. When I program my water drinking into the day and carry it with me, I inevitably feel much better.

In your *Stripped* menu plan you will drink 500 ml or two cups of water at each of your five or six daily meals. If you are hungry between meals or after your last meal, drink water. Staying hydrated also reduces food cravings and suppresses the appetite. Avoid juice and flavor crystals – these are packed with sugar and fake sugar. Kick up the flavor level of your water with a squeeze of fresh lemon. (See more *Stripped* drink recipes on page 158.)

> "Water is second only to oxygen in the level of importance it has to the body."

7 Carry a cooler packed with Clean foods each day.

Having your meals ready to eat at the beginning of each day and taking them with you is key to success when Eating Clean. It's easy enough to Eat Clean at home with a full refrigerator, pantry and kitchen stocked with cooking gadgets. As soon as you step out your front door it becomes a much more difficult task.

If you want to be completely aware of what kind of fuel you're putting into your body at all times, you must prepare your food at home and take it with you. Do you know how the salad at your favorite restaurant was prepared? Can you be sure that the soup at your local deli wasn't made with excess oils and heavy creams?

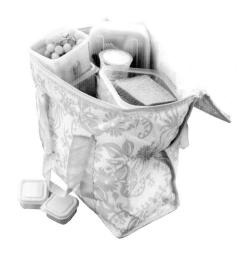

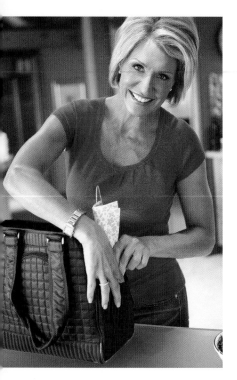

▲ **PACKING MY COOLER** each day puts me in a position to succeed. It's optimization at work!

Purchase a cooler that has a sturdy handle and is large enough to carry at least three Clean meals at a time. If you work a typical nine to five day job, you'll eat your breakfast at home, your next three meals out of the house, and your dinner and evening meals at home. When you carry your meals with you, it's easy to eat every three hours on schedule and you won't be tempted by hunger and stray off plan.

To make it easier on yourself, get into the habit of making more food than you need for one meal and using it to pack the next day's cooler. When you grill chicken breasts, make five or six instead of just one. Boil a big pot of brown rice at the beginning of the week. Instead of chopping just one pepper, chop two peppers, your carrots and celery, etc. When you have Clean food ready to go, packing your cooler is a breeze!

In your *Stripped* meal plan, you'll need to make your own food and take it with you to ensure success. I like to pack my cooler the night before. It's no stress in the morning – I just grab it and go.

8 Depend on fresh fruits and vegetables for fiber, vitamins, nutrients and enzymes.

Eating Clean is not just about losing weight. It's definitely a huge benefit, yes, but you also Eat Clean to improve your health and this is where fruits and vegetables come in. If your current diet does not include a large variety of these delicious natural wonders, be prepared to widen your palate. To get rid of your last 10 pounds in a healthy way, without depriving yourself and sacrificing nutrition, you must supplement your diet with an abundance of fruits and veggies. As an added benefit your health will experience a positive boost too!

It may be strange to think of fruits and vegetables as carbohydrates. The low-carb diet craze has tainted our minds into thinking that carbohydrates come from only starchy sources such as bread and pasta. A better approach to thinking about carbs is to acknowledge they come in two very different groups: simple carbohydrates found in sugar and refined foods, and complex carbohydrates found in whole grains, fruits and vegetables.

Complex carbohydrates from fruits and vegetables contain much-needed vitamins, nutrients and enzymes. They take their time being processed in your stomach and keep your blood-sugar levels stable, which is the reason you feel full and your energy stays constant between meals.

In your *Stripped* meal plan, you will eat fruit, vegetables or both at each of your five or six daily meals.

ALLOWABLE VEGETABLES INCLUDE:
Sweet and regular potatoes, radishes, carrots, parsnips, cucumber, broccoli, asparagus, beets, leeks, leafy greens, Brussels sprouts, green beans, onions, sprouts, celery, zucchini, fennel and garlic.

ALLOWABLE FRUITS INCLUDE:
Bananas, apples, plums, berries, pears, watermelon, cherries, oranges, tomatoes, limes and lemons.

"To get rid of your last 10 pounds in a healthy way, without depriving yourself and sacrificing nutrition, you must supplement your diet with an abundance of fruits and veggies."

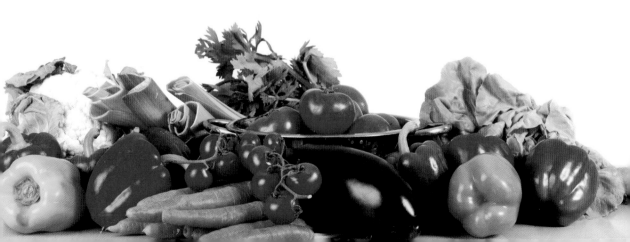

A "HANDY" GUIDE

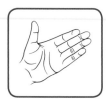

Protein

A proper portion of meat or other protein is measured by what can fit into the palm of one hand.

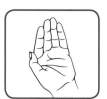

Starchy Complex Carbohydrates

A proper portion of starchy carbs is measured by what can fit into one cupped hand.

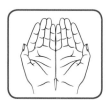

Carbs from Fruits and Vegetables

A proper portion of complex carbohydrates from fresh produce is measured by what can fit into two hands cupped together.

Healthy Fats

A portion of healthy fats is one scant handful of nuts, or one to two tablespoons of healthy oil or nut butter.

9 Adhere to proper portion sizes

Now that you are eating five or six meals every day, you are going to have to eat smaller amounts of food at each sitting. You'll still feel satisfied – trust me. If anything, you'll be amazed at the amount of food you get to eat. Initially, you will feel as if you are getting away with something. When I first started Eating Clean, I couldn't believe that I could get away with eating so much while watching my size get smaller. It seemed too good to be true!

Eating Clean works because you eat the right amount of food for your specific body size. Think about it – a burly 6'5" man would need a heck of a lot more food to survive than a petite 5'2" woman. Everyone cannot eat similar portion sizes and expect to maintain their weight – it's just not realistic. This is one of the reasons women tend to gain weight during long-term relationships with men. They slowly increase their portions to match that of their partners's and the result is tighter pants and a higher number on the scale.

In your *Stripped* meal plan, the amount of food you will eat depends on the size of your hands. This is the only tool you need to determine how much food is the right amount of food for your body. Use the guide on the left to help you measure out your portions of protein, starchy complex carbohydrates, complex carbohydrates from fruits and vegetables, and healthy fats. If you would like to measure your food in cups and grams, use your hands the first time and pour that amount into the measuring system you prefer. I stick to using my hands as a guide because it's simple and I know I'll always have them ... on hand.

10 Eat only foods that have not been overly processed or doused in chemicals, saturated and trans fats and/or toxins.

I like to divide all foods into two major categories: real foods and "anti" foods. What do I mean by this? Real foods are those found in nature. They often have only one ingredient such as oats, apples, broccoli or brown rice. Real foods are not altered in any way and nothing is added to make them taste better – they taste best on their own. "Anti" foods are foods that have been altered or overly processed – most of these come in the form of prepackaged food products such as Twinkies, crackers, candy and white bread.

Real foods give you the most nutritional bang for your buck. Eating nutrient-dense foods makes an enormous and notable difference both in your health and your physique. These are the foods that fuel your body, keep your blood-sugar levels stable and

"Eating nutrient-dense foods makes an enormous and notable difference both in your health and your physique."

> "The cardinal rule for Eating Clean is: the fewer ingredients on the label, the better."

your hunger at bay between meals. It is very difficult to lose or maintain your weight without depending on real foods for your meal choices.

Foods with added sugars, trans fats or made with processed white grains and flours can cause a spike in insulin levels, which in turn makes your metabolism slow down. It's also common to feel hungry shortly after eating these "anti" foods, because they don't contain the nutrients your body needs to feel satiated.

If you are in doubt as to which foods are "real" and which are "anti" foods, read the ingredient list and nutrition label. The cardinal rule for Eating Clean is: the fewer ingredients on the label, the better. Foods with one ingredient, as I mentioned before, should be your top choice. If the product you are thinking of choosing contains ingredients you've never heard of or can't pronounce, leave it on the shelf.

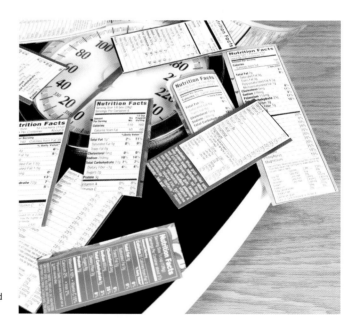

▶ **GET IN THE HABIT** of reading the ingredients list on every packaged food item you purchase.

Summary:

THE EAT-CLEAN DIET PRINCIPLES

1 Eat more! Eat six small meals each day, spaced at two-and-a-half to three-hour intervals.

2 Eat breakfast every day, within an hour of rising.

3 Make your last meal three hours before bed.

4 Eat a combination of lean protein and complex carbohydrates at each meal.

5 Eat sufficient healthy fats every day.

6 Drink two to three liters of water each day.

7 Carry a cooler packed with Clean foods each day.

8 Depend on fresh fruits and vegetables for fiber, vitamins, nutrients and enzymes.

9 Adhere to proper portion sizes.

10 Eat only foods that have not been overly processed or doused in chemicals, saturated and trans fats and/or toxins.

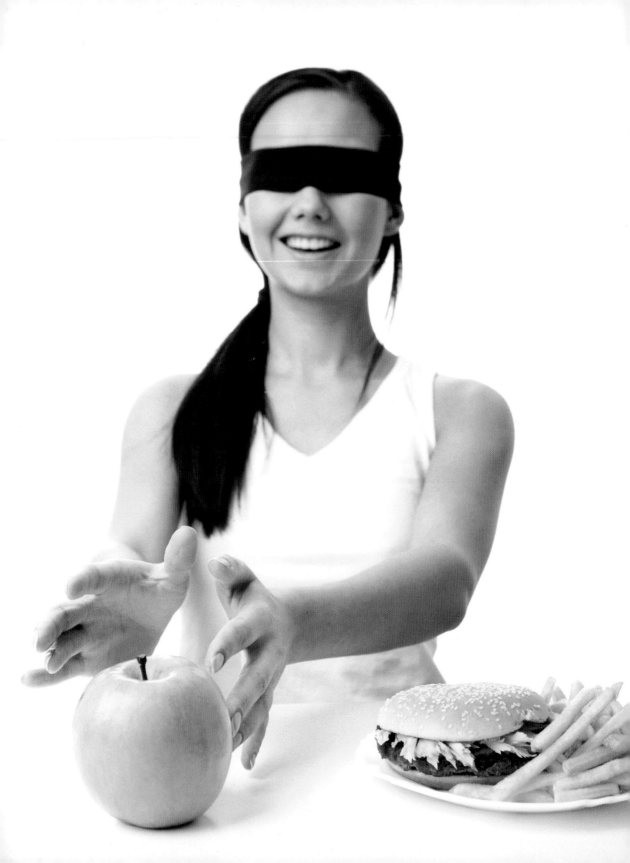

5 | Food Versus "Anti" Food

Y ou now know the 10 *Eat-Clean Diet* Principles. If you doubt that food choices can be more effective in overhauling your physique than a fad diet, pill or surgical procedure, chew on this: with sales of the *Eat-Clean Diet* series in the millions, a great many of you have changed your lives by switching from being a mindless eater to a mindful eater.

> Much of what we do to burn away the final 10 pounds relies on consuming foods that are natural, unprocessed and loaded with nutrients.

The diet works because the Principles are logical, simple and effective. It makes sense to eschew all processed foods or those filled with sugar and trans fats because we didn't have them throughout history. Our Creator sowed the earth with plant material and other organisms to offer nutrition. All that has changed now. What was once the simple act of eating is now a minefield of trouble. Much of what we do to burn away the final 10 pounds relies on consuming foods that are natural, unprocessed and loaded with nutrients.

The Macronutrients

Forget fad diets that tell you to avoid all fats and the other sorts that tell you to load up on only protein. These tricks don't have legs. You want a way of eating that will help you kick your weight problem once and for all. No one can survive on meat, meat and more meat for very long. This sort of fad-diet eating does not help you fix even a 10-pound weight problem for good; it's only for the short haul, and then what kind of damage are you doing to your metabolism and your health? And how does a person really function on zero carbohydrates? I have tried it myself. It is impossible and, I believe, dangerous. When I don't eat carbs I can hardly operate a telephone, let alone a car.

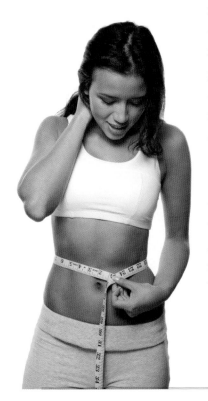

The Eat-Clean Diet Stripped is based on eating whole foods from all the most nutritious food groups including protein, complex carbohydrates from fresh fruits and vegetables and from whole grains. We don't ignore healthy fats, either. Without them your metabolism nosedives and your nervous system, including your brain function, is placed at risk.

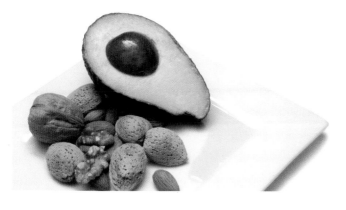

The abundance of nutrient-dense foods that will make up the backbone of your eating in the 28 days to come and for the rest of your life will not only transform your body, but also your health. Each of the five or six meals you will be eating each day from now on can be viewed as an opportunity to load up your body with health-boosting fat-blasting nutrients. Proteins, plants, grains and fats are the macronutrients needed to create the most vital version of you possible. Embrace these as the gold standard of foods for your weight-loss plan. Accept no others!

Protein: The Building Material You Need for Weight Control

Muscle is the most metabolically active tissue in the body. It is the most abundant (unless you are obese) as well. And here is the best news for you, the person who wants to lose weight: Muscle is the hungriest tissue in your body. If muscle tissue is hungry, it makes sense that the more of it you have, the faster your metabolism will burn. Now you are getting it! Building a layer of lean muscle on your frame is the way to launch your metabolism into high gear. This is one of the goals of your *Stripped* plan – building a beautiful body with lean muscle.

Once we have that muscle, how do we feed it? The best food for muscle is protein. The reason for this is that protein contains amino acids, which are the building blocks of muscle tissue and all other tissues in the body. Protein is needed to repair and build these tissues. This is one of the reasons protein is included at each of the five or six meals eaten every day in *The Eat-Clean Diet*. Dietary protein also stimulates the fat-burning hormone called glucagon, activating it to do its job. Protein is also a "thermogenic" food, which is a fancy way of saying it turns up our furnace to burn unwanted body fat.

There are two main kinds of thermogenesis: one happens when you move or shiver (exercise-induced thermogenesis) and the other happens when you eat. Have you ever noticed after eating you begin to feel sweaty and hot? This is food-induced thermogenesis. Basically, your body needs more energy to digest what you just ate. The harder it is for your body to digest a food, the more thermogenic it is.

"The best food for muscle is protein. The reason for this is that protein contains amino acids, which are the building blocks of muscle tissue and all other tissues in the body."

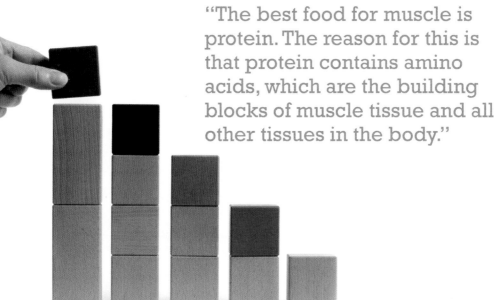

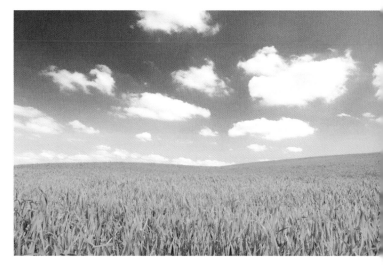

Learning how to take advantage of the thermic effect of certain foods will help you lose those last 10 pounds. The combination of lean protein and complex carbohydrates I advocate eating in this *Stripped* plan is the way to do this. While you are eating these foods you are nourishing yourself but also burning extra fuel in order to digest them.

The key is learning to identify optimal protein sources for your new body. Big Macs won't cut it. You need the best sources of lean and nutritious protein on your plate. The better the quality of protein you eat, the faster you will drop a dress size. That should encourage you to make better protein choices! Consider such excellent options as organic eggs, grass-fed beef, bison and poultry. Wild game is also excellent because the meat is not tainted with chemicals and hormones. Grass-fed animals are often healthier and happier while having a denser nutritional profile. I also love goat's milk and yogurt. Goat's milk is very high in readily digestible protein and is better tolerated by those with lactose intolerance. Although dairy is not included in your *Stripped* meal plan, it can be a great addition to your weight-maintenance plan.

"Grass-fed animals are often healthier and happier while having a denser nutritional profile."

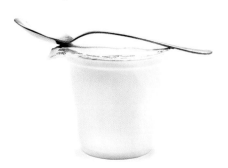

◀ **DAIRY CAN BE** an excellent source of protein for both meat eaters and vegetarians alike.

Next you will discover the optimum timing of feeding those hungry muscles is every three hours. That means you will be eating some kind of protein at each of your five or six daily meals. You will quickly become accustomed to this practice as the days go by. Most of us can absorb only about 20 grams of protein at one serving. If you are measuring protein powder there is normally a convenient scoop included in the package. When it comes to meat and other protein foods I have devised a handy way of working out how much is right for you. Using a finger, trace out the palm on one hand. The size of one of your palms will be the correct amount of protein to eat at a meal. If you are eating tofu, then check the serving size and protein amount on the package. Be careful with nuts; they are an excellent source of protein and other nutrients, but they are high in fat. Although these are healthy fats, you don't want to overdo them. I know I'm repeating myself here, but measure out a quarter-cup of nuts and put the rest away. I count out about 12 almonds along with two Brazil nuts and that's my limit for the day. Egg whites are easy too. One egg white contains about five grams of protein, so you will need to eat four to get your 20 grams.

PROTEIN AT-A-GLANCE

How does protein help you drop 10 pounds and feel fantastic?

→ Protein stabilizes blood sugar levels.

→ Protein strengthens and maintains your immune system.

→ Protein enhances cell metabolism thus increasing your metabolic rate.

→ Protein helps build lean muscle tissue increasing your metabolic rate.

→ Protein encourages hormone production, in particular glucagon.

→ Protein balances body fluids.

→ Protein promotes enzyme production.

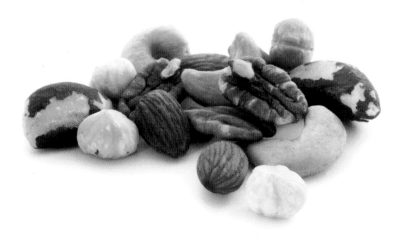

IF YOU ARE AGAINST EATING ANIMALS or animal products you should consider eating quinoa. This superfood is actually the seed of a flowering plant, so it is gluten free and great for celiacs but considered a grain. In ancient Mayan times this grain essentially supported an entire civilization. The Mayas called quinoa the "mother grain" so highly did they prize this food.

A one-cup serving of quinoa contains eight grams of readily digestible protein – that's twice the amount you will find in any other grain. Quinoa is also a complete protein, which means it contains all nine essential amino acids the body requires for optimum health. Quinoa also contains excellent quantities of numerous vitamins and minerals including: iron, calcium, potassium, zinc, vitamin E, selenium, magnesium, manganese, tryptophan, copper, phosphorus and fiber.

Remember to rinse your quinoa grains well before cooking to remove the bitter coating. And then eat quinoa sweet or savory! I love it as a side dish, particularly in the summer when I can make up a savory quinoa salad in the morning, refrigerate it and serve it for dinner with sliced summer vegetables. Delicious!

HOW TO COOK QUINOA

1. **RINSE QUINOA well in a fine mesh sieve or strainer. Quinoa has an unpleasant, bitter taste if this step is skipped.**

NOTE: *Quinoa needs to cook in a ratio of one part quinoa to one-and-three-quarters part liquid. If you are cooking one cup of uncooked quinoa, you need one and three-quarters of a cup of water.*

2. **BRING LIQUID to a boil over high heat, then add uncooked quinoa and stir until mixed.**

3. **LOWER HEAT to a simmer and cook uncovered for 12 to 15 minutes, until all liquid is absorbed. Fluff with a fork and serve.**

NOTE: *You can change the taste of your quinoa by cooking it in various liquids, from water to broth to cranberry juice.*

"Remember to rinse your quinoa grains well before cooking to remove the bitter coating."

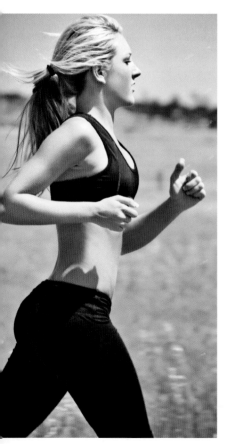

> "The foods you choose impact your metabolism. The effect you would most like to see is an increased metabolic rate."

How Does Food Alter Your Metabolism?

Your body has a system for burning fuel called the metabolism. This system also burns fat already on your body. The metabolism is a lot like the heating system in your house. If you put good fuel into the furnace it will produce heat, keeping you warm, comfortable and even happy. If you put poor-quality or insufficient fuel into the furnace, you will be cold, tired, lacking energy and you will feel miserable. If you feed yourself with nutrient-dense foods at regular intervals your body will produce energy, and keep you warm and energetic. If you feed yourself nutritionally empty foods your body will respond with a slower metabolism, poor circulation, weight gain, diminished energy levels, fatigue and a host of problems that spell disaster.

The foods you choose impact your metabolism. The effect you would most like to see is an increased metabolic rate. Food does this through the various phytochemicals (plant nutrients) they contain and also through their chemical makeup. Imagine, for example, a chicken breast. The protein in the chicken breast takes a considerable amount of energy just to break down. When you eat sugary treats or even drink a glass of orange juice, it breaks down very easily, spiking your blood sugar instead of your metabolism.

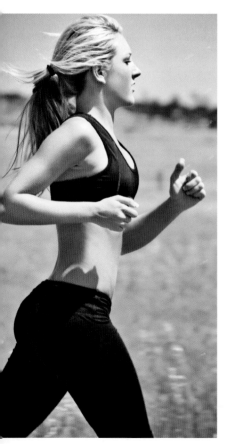

YOUR METABOLIC RATE (the speed of your metabolism) is determined by several factors, including your genetics, the food you eat, your height and weight, your muscle mass and your activity level. By changing your lifestyle, you can speed up your metabolism and lose weight without struggling. You don't have to become a marathon runner, but you do have to get up off the couch and make the following changes:

① Start training with weights.

You need to build muscle to burn fat. One pound of muscle burns far more calories than a pound of fat. And strength training not only stimulates your muscles while you're working out, but for hours afterwards.

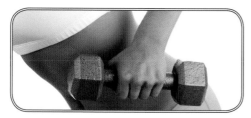

② Get moving!

Increase the intensity (not the duration) of your cardio workouts. To make the most of your heart-pumping workouts, try HIIT (high-intensity interval training). Studies show that people who incorporate HIIT into their workouts lose twice as much weight as those who don't.

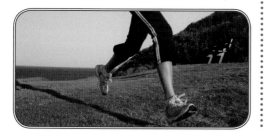

③ Eat regularly.

Eating small meals every two-and-a-half to three hours ensures your metabolism will stay hyped all day long. When you wait too long between meals or skip one entirely, you trigger a starvation response and your metabolism begins to slow down.

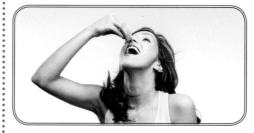

④ Drink plenty of water.

We often confuse thirst for hunger and this is easily preventable by keeping a loaded water bottle nearby. Drinking water also keeps your body lean by helping nutrients flow through it, and by washing away waste and free radicals.

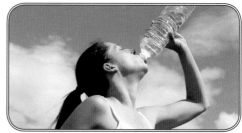

Unrefined Carbohydrates

QUESTION: When is sugar not a poison?

ANSWER: When it's natural and comes with fiber.

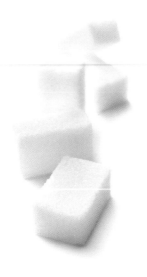

An enormous amount of confusion is associated with carbohydrates. This is partly because of low-carb fad diets and partly thanks to nutrition labels. Unfortunately sugar, including the white processed stuff we pour on everything, is lumped in with good carbohydrates including those we get from eating fresh fruits and vegetables as well as whole grains. So when we see the sugar content on a nutrition label it is easy to become confused and think that food is full of added sugars, when it may not be. Check the ingredient list, and then think of carbohydrates as one of two kinds: either refined or unrefined.

A refined carbohydrate such as white table sugar will almost immediately turn to glucose, the preferred fuel in your body, as soon as you eat it. It will cause your pancreas to release a flood of insulin, your blood's manager of glucose.

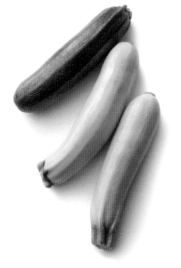

Unrefined carbohydrates, on the other hand, contain not just nutritional value and plant sugars, but fiber as well. It is the presence of fiber that mitigates the effect of plant-based carbohydrates in the blood. Fiber takes a lot of work to process because it is indigestible. Therefore its presence slows down the release of glucose into the blood, helping to keep insulin levels even and you slim!

Unrefined carbohydrates from fruits and vegetables as well as whole grains are the ideal foods for you to eat, partnered with lean protein. This is the optimum fuel to run the everyday workings of your human engine. A sports car such as a Ferrari performs optimally on high-octane fuel, and your body also performs best on nutrient-dense fuel.

Healthy Fats

Don't worry – fats are not a four-letter word! You and I absolutely need good fats in our bodies even though we might be trying to lose 10 pounds. Fat is part of our physical makeup. We have quite a lot of fat in our brains – approximately 60 percent of our noodle is fat. Each of the trillions of cells in our body is covered in fat. It's also in our eyes and ears, and in our sex and adrenal glands. It's everywhere, so embrace it. The fat you want to be rid of is that layer around your middle and on your butt. We are going to do something about this fat!

"You and I absolutely need good fats in our bodies even though we might be trying to lose 10 pounds. Fat is part of our physical makeup."

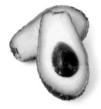

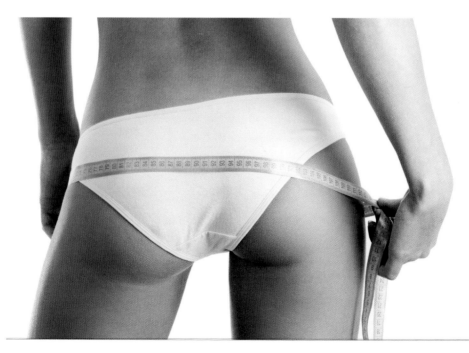

FATS – THE GOOD GUYS

What can healthy fats do to help you lose weight?

→ Fortify cell walls

→ Balance blood-sugar levels

→ Provide fuel for long-term energy

→ Provide the building materials needed to make hormones

FATS – THE BAD GUYS

→ Trans fats

→ Saturated fats – an excess of saturated fats from animal products

→ Man-made fats as in margarine

Healthy fats found in fish, seeds, nuts and plants are bound to help you increase your metabolic rate and your energy levels. Could your weight problem be related to something as simple as fat? Indeed! You need to eat omega-6 and omega-3 fatty acids in the right balance, which most experts suggest is something between 1:1 and 4:1. Translated, that means you should be eating a maximum of four parts omega-6 to one part omega-3. It may surprise you to learn that the Standard American Diet (SAD) is skewed much too far in the direction of omega-6 fatty acids. The ratio looks something like 50:1, which is shocking and that is one reason we are tired, fat and sick.

How does fat burn fat? These fatty acids work together to make our trillions of cells use more oxygen, which increases the cells' ability to produce energy. The more oxygen our cells use, the more energy they produce and the faster our metabolism works, meaning we burn more fat. You see how marvelous this is? You really do have a fighting chance to finally burn away the last 10 pounds and fat is one part of the solution.

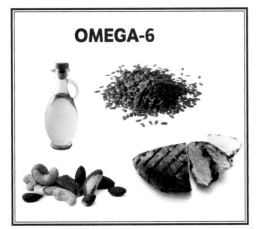

OMEGA-6

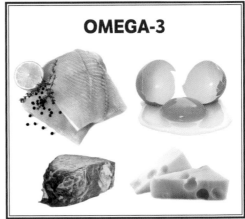

OMEGA-3

EATING CLEAN – WHAT TO AVOID

Here is your list of Eat-Clean no-nos. Stay away from these things – they will not help you lose those last 10 pounds.

1 All refined, over-processed foods, particularly white flour, sugar and related products.

2 Chemically charged foods.

3 Foods containing preservatives.

4 Saturated and trans fats.

5 Skipping meals.

6 Excess sodium.

7 Sugar and all sugar substitutes.

8 Counting calories.

9 Alcohol and juice – both beverages are packed with sugar!

10 Artificial foods.

11 All calorie-dense foods containing little or no nutritional value. I call these "anti" foods.

12 Supersizing your meals.

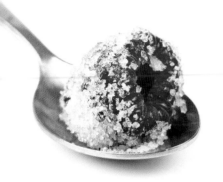

Sugar: The Ultimate "Anti" Food

"It is quite possible to improve your disposition, increase your efficiency and change your personality for the better. The way to do it is to avoid cane and beet sugar in all forms and guises." – Dr. John W. Tintera

If you decide to do just the bare minimum and nothing else, I urge you to follow these Eat-Clean Diet Principles: Eat only foods that have not been overly processed or doused in chemicals, saturated and trans fats and/or toxins, and **do not eat processed food, especially sugar and white flour.**

> "The white crystalline powder is so ubiquitous we can no longer recognize the flavor of food without it. I rank sugar's dangerous effects up there with cocaine and heroin."

Sugar is white poison. We have been assaulted by this "anti" food as it has steadily crept into everything that touches our lips, from cigarettes to salt, processed meats, medicine and more. It has done us no good. As surely as our safety has been threatened by terrorism, so too has our health been attacked by this evil "anti" food. The white crystalline powder is so ubiquitous we can no longer recognize the flavor of food without it. I rank sugar's dangerous effects up there with cocaine and heroin. All three are white powders, all give you a high and crushing lows, all are highly addictive and all destroy you. Sugar may be even more dangerous because it is legal and so we are not prepared for its disastrous effects.

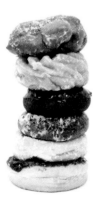

I am not overstating the situation. From the beginning of time until the 1800s we ate almost no sugar. Then in less than 100 years we jumped to an average 60 pounds of sugar per person per year, or one pound every few days. And some consume much more. The bulk of this sugar comes from soda and fruit juices. In the days of Adam refined sugar was never part of the human diet. People ate what grew naturally from the soil or hung from trees – fruit, nuts, dates, apples, figs, grains, legumes, milk and honey. As William Dufty says in one of my favorite books on the subject of sugar, *Sugar Blues*, "… sugar was unknown to man." The Greeks, from whence came our modern alphabet, had no word for sugar.

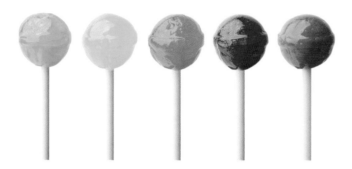

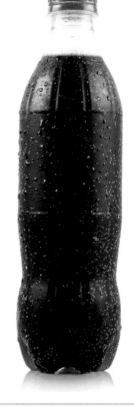

▼ **IF SUGAR** is on the ingredients list of a packaged food, that means it's added and not natural.

When I tell people to stop eating refined sugar in all its disguises, their faces express unabashed horror. I guess I shouldn't be surprised, as I have seen young mothers put Orange Crush soda in their infant's baby bottle. I helped a man regain his life by doing nothing more than getting him to quit his 12-Coke-a-day habit. He had been drinking this for years and was obese (at least 100 pounds overweight), wore headgear to bed for his sleep apnea, had diabetes, hypertension, no libido, severe headaches, terrible skin and was interminably exhausted, all at the young age of 26. Simply exchanging Coke (sugar) for water helped him shed his excess weight. He was able to run a marathon, wear normal-sized clothing and get positive marks on his health check-up. He was even interested in being with his wife in a loving way again, which would be much more fun without that annoying headgear!

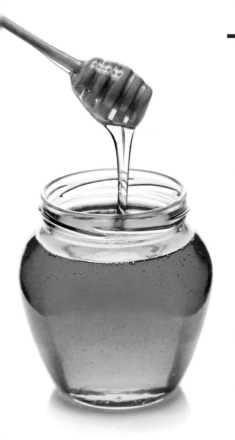

> "Once you are maintaining your weight loss you can have an occasional treat, but for now you should avoid all sweeteners."

Beware the Fakes!

Let me caution you not to exchange one poison for another. If you're tempted to load up on artificial sweeteners, don't go there! They are equally detrimental to your health and your weight-loss goals. People often ask me about stevia. For now I say it's okay to use the real stuff, but please use your own judgment. And watch out for fake stevia, too! Once you are maintaining your weight loss you can have an occasional treat, but for now you should avoid all sweeteners.

The following boxes will help you recognize sugar (it has a lot of names!) and the many forms of fake sugar:

SUGAR – RECOGNIZE ITS MANY FORMS

→ Agave nectar
→ Barbados sugar
→ Barley malt
→ Beet sugar
→ Blackstrap molasses
→ Brown sugar
→ Cane crystals
→ Cane sugar
→ Caramel
→ Carob syrup
→ Confectioners sugar
→ Corn syrup
→ Date sugar
→ Demerara sugar

→ Dextrin
→ Dextrose
→ Evaporated cane juice
→ Ethyl maltol
→ Fructose
→ Fruit juice
→ Fruit juice concentrate
→ Galactose
→ Glucose
→ Golden sugar
→ Golden syrup
→ Granulated sugar
→ Grape sugar
→ Grape juice concentrate

- → High-fructose corn syrup/ HFCS
- → Honey
- → Icing sugar
- → Invert sugar
- → Lactose
- → Malt syrup
- → Maltodextrin
- → Maltose
- → Maple syrup
- → Molasses
- → Moscovado sugar
- → Organic raw sugar
- → Powdered sugar
- → Raw sugar
- → Rice syrup
- → Sorbitol
- → Sorghum syrup
- → Sucrose
- → Sugar
- → Table sugar
- → Treacle
- → Turbinado sugar
- → Yellow sugar

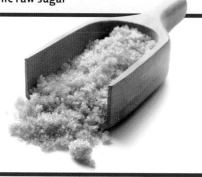

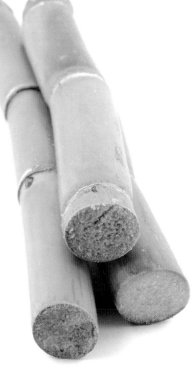

▲ ALCOHOL (RUM), ROCK CANDY, molasses and syrups are all products of the sugar cane plant.

ARTIFICIAL SWEETENERS – THE FAKES

- → Acesulfame K
- → Alitame
- → Aspartame (NutraSweet, Equal)
- → Cyclamate (lost its FDA approval in 1970 but is being reconsidered)
- → Neotame
- → Saccharin
- → Sucralose (Splenda)
- → Sweetener blend: containing a combination of aspartame, sucralose & acesulfame K

> "Learning to recognize the enemy will help us win the battle against the last 10 pounds clinging to our waists and it will foster improved health."

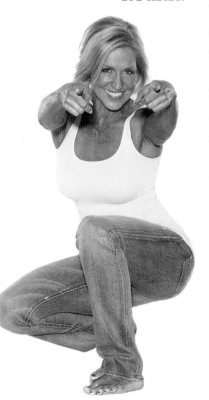

Give Up On Sugar

So many food products contain some form of sugar, sugar alternative or sweetener, it is almost impossible for us to keep up with figuring out whether a food is Clean or not. This is one of the reasons I strongly urge you to become familiar with this deadly ingredient and avoid it altogether. Another compelling reason is that the human body is simply not designed to keep up with this deluge of sugar. We are losing the battle, as millions of North Americans are now diabetic, pre-diabetic or afflicted with disease. Sugar lives among us but we do not see it, nor do we comprehend that there are thousands of vendors of sugar-infested foods and other "anti" foods that are keenly interested in swamping us with the stuff so we become addicted. If the flow of White Poison is not dammed, not only will humanity become cripplingly ill at a faster and faster pace, but we will also bankrupt the health care system and ourselves as we go.

Learning to recognize the enemy will help us win the battle against the last 10 pounds clinging to our waists and it will foster improved health.

The antidote to sugar-laden, nutrient-devoid foods is to eat whole, Clean, nourishing foods in their most natural and unprocessed state. What follows is health and wellness like nothing you have experienced before. It is the way we have always been intended to eat. Nothing could be simpler or more truthful for you. Nothing will help you change your body more dramatically.

"What we call diseases and illnesses are merely symptoms that the entire body is out of kilter. To make a man whole again he has only to eat whole food." - William Dufty, *Sugar Blues*.

YOUR CHOICE TO EAT CLEAN contributes positively to the greening of our planet. Many of us blindly select food (even Clean food) without considering its effect on the earth. By Eating Clean you are helping the environment by making informed food decisions and reducing your carbon footprint. How? Take the time to think about the following global issues.

Fresh Fruit and Vegetables

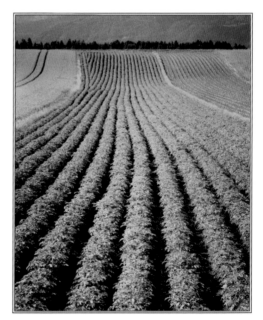

The Eat-Clean Diet promotes fresh foods over processed foods. Purchasing fresh foods means far less packaging. This in turn reduces the amount of air pollution, landfill waste and energy consumption. When you take into account the greenhouse gases emitted to create the paper, plastic and metal packaging for processed foods, the energy consumed to power these factories and the garbage left behind, it's easy to see why fresh is better. But even fresh produce has to be considered before purchase. The more miles your food is transported, whether by land, sea or air, the larger the carbon footprint. The solution is to buy locally grown produce. Purchasing local foods encourages you to buy in season, which is when produce is freshest, has a higher nutritional value and is also lighter on your wallet. As a bonus, you help your local economy.

Meat and Poultry

Organic is the most environmentally friendly way to go. Non-organic farming accumulates an overabundance of livestock waste, leading to unhealthy amounts of methane and other harmful pollutants. Large-scale cattle ranching is a key player in the deforestation of the Amazon, contributing to a fifth of global greenhouse gas emissions.[i] Organic farms house fewer livestock, decreasing the amount of waste produced, and virtually eliminating disease and infection in animals. Allowing livestock to range freely is a more humane way to raise living creatures, which is healthier for the animals, the humans consuming them and the ecosystems surrounding them.

FOR THE MOST PART, USDA ORGANIC LABEL DENOTES THAT:

→ The farmer has not used antibiotics or synthetic growth hormones.

→ The farmer has fed with 100% organic feed.

→ Animals are given access to the outdoors and/or pastures.

→ The farmer has not used most conventional pesticides, synthetic fertilizers, bioengineering or ionizing radiation.

→ There is an emphasis on renewable resources and conservation at the farm.

The organic product industry has not been fully regulated and unruly business practices do exist. It is ultimately up to the consumer to make informed selections when selecting meat and poultry and choose a trusted source.

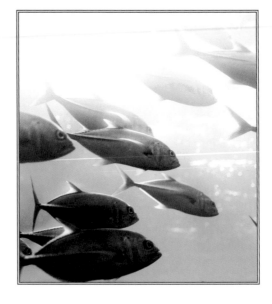

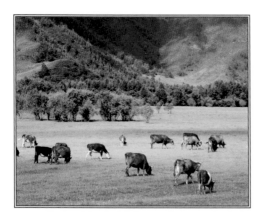

Fish

Fish is an ideal source of protein, but we must be mindful of where and how fish is being farmed or caught. Overfishing leads to ecological imbalances. To help make wiser seafood choices, here is a reference list of the 15 most destructively fished or farmed species based on stock status, habitat impacts, destructive fishing methods, illegal fishing, poor management and social impacts. Do not purchase or order these types of fish. If you feel so inclined you can let your local restaurants and supermarkets know that these are environmentally sensitive species and suggest that they cease their distribution and order alternative options. But do it with a smile!

AVOID THESE FISH[ii]

→ Atlantic haddock

→ Atlantic cod

→ Atlantic halibut

→ Atlantic salmon (farmed)

→ Atlantic sea scallops

→ Chilean sea bass

→ Greenland halibut

→ Hard shell clams

→ New Zealand hoki

→ Orange roughy

→ Sharks

→ Skates and rays

→ Swordfish

→ Tropical shrimps

→ Tuna – blue fin, big eye, yellow fin

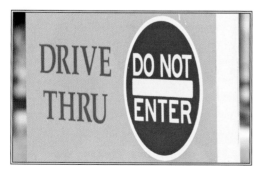

Fast-Food Industry

When you Eat Clean you automatically reduce the number of visits to fast-food establishments. This alone decreases the amount of waste from packaging. A drive thru is convenient, but as a follower of the Eat-Clean Diet lifestyle you will learn that everything "convenient" in the food world bears consequences. The drive-thru window is one of the worst contributors to your carbon footprint as a result of the emissions produced from idling cars as well as garbage. Think of how long you idle your car in a drive-thru line-up – anywhere from two to ten minutes. "For every two minutes a car is idling, it uses about the same amount of fuel it takes to go about one mile."[iii] If you must stop at a fast-food chain or coffee shop, park your car, walk in and make a healthy food selection. Chances are you will be in and out faster than you would have in that busy drive-thru line-up.

Eating Clean and being well informed about your food choices will not only create a healthier you, it offers the necessary steps toward shaping a healthier planet, too. When shopping at your local supermarket for Clean food, always remember to ask yourself how and where your food was grown, raised, picked, caught, transported and sold. And don't forget your reusable bags!

i http://www.greenpeace.org/international/en/news/features/cattle-mapping/
ii http://www.greenpeace.org/canada/campaigns/Seafood/Get-involved/redlist/
iii http://www.consumerenergycenter.org/myths/idling.html

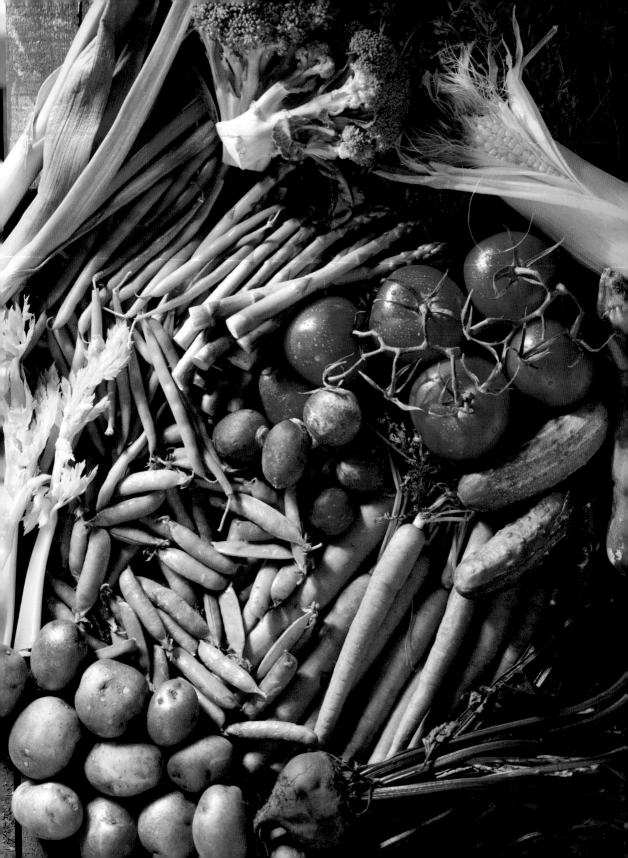

6 | *Stripped* *Vegetarian Style*

Following the Eat-Clean lifestyle as a vegetarian is simple. You must ensure you include protein-rich plant foods at each of your five or six daily meals. If you eat eggs and fish, it's easier still. But you will find it a little tougher when trying to lose those last 10 pounds. Vegetarians tend to get a lot of their calories from starchy sources, and on the *Stripped* plan you will have to be more mindful of your consumption of these foods.

"Seek out protein in everything from your greens to your grains."

Vegetarian Sources of Protein

If you are a lacto-ovo vegetarian then you'll have to forget the "lacto" while following the *Eat-Clean Diet Stripped* plan, but you can eat plenty of "ovos," focusing on the whites only, however. The only real limit on the number of egg whites you should consume is the number you feel comfortable eating – meaning your appetite and your abdomen, since some people find eggs give them gas. Also remember that the body can process only about 20 grams of protein at one time. One egg white contains five grams of protein – you can do the math.

The key to weight-loss success is to conscientiously take in as much protein as possible throughout your diet. In other words, you should seek out protein in everything from your greens to your grains. Contributing to the challenge, you'll have to avoid starchy high-protein sources such as most beans. Beans are often the go-to food for vegetarians, so you'll have to put some careful thought into your food choices each day. You'll also have to avoid foods high in natural sugars, such as dairy. If you are not a vegan, chances are you rely on dairy products for your protein, but this category is off limits when losing those very stubborn last 10 pounds.

Eat High-Protein Vegetables

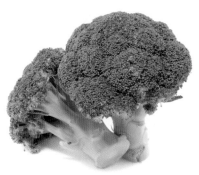

You may be surprised to learn that there are numerous plants, and by extension vegetables, that contain significant amounts of protein. By high-protein vegetables, I don't mean plant-based protein sources; I mean actual vegetables. Sea vegetables contain especially large amounts of protein. Blue-green algae, such as spirulina, are an incredible source of protein, with one mere tablespoon (dried) containing four grams. Seaweeds such as nori, the seaweed used to wrap sushi, are another good protein source.

Most cruciferous vegetables are fairly high in protein. Broccoli, Brussels sprouts, cauliflower and asparagus each contain about three grams of protein per 100 grams. Spinach, surprisingly, contains equal amounts of protein and carbohydrate, with no fat. While its relatives kale and Swiss chard cannot boast the same, they do still have substantial amounts of protein. Most beans and lentils will have too much starch for your *Stripped* eating plan, but bean sprouts are high in protein and highly nutritious in general. A similar food, watercress, also contains considerable protein.

These vegetable sources of protein are not complete (meaning they do not offer a full array of essential amino acids), and I do not suggest them as your main protein source, but making sure you have a serving of one of these vegetables at each of your daily meals will really help you get in your protein without relying on foods that won't help you achieve your goals.

High-Protein Grains

You may know that oatmeal is one of my favorite foods – with good reason! This grain is chock-full of nutrition and even contains a considerable amount of protein. Your other high-protein grain option is quinoa. Actually a seed rather than a grain, the superfood quinoa contains protein and healthy fats along with its carbohydrates. Unlike most plant-based protein foods, quinoa contains all the essential amino acids in adequate numbers, and is therefore considered a complete protein.

Soy

Most beans and lentils are too high in starchy carbohydrates for you to eat at this time as a protein source; the exception is soy. It is about one-third protein, and that makes soy and soy products

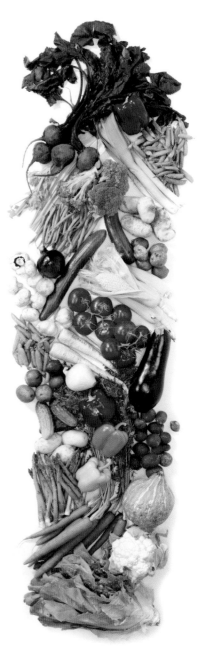

Vegetarian Protein Source Guide

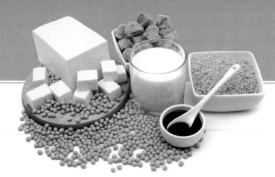

WITH THIS HELPFUL GUIDE, you'll be able to figure out the protein in a standard serving of your favorite vegetarian sources.

Source	Serving	Protein
Egg whites	4 whites	20 g protein
Algae (spirulina)	2 Tbsp / 480 ml	8 g protein
Seaweed (nori)	10 sheets	2 g protein
Broccoli	2 cups / 480 ml	6 g protein
Brussels sprouts	2 cups / 480 ml	6 g protein
Cauliflower	2 cups / 480 ml	4 g protein
Asparagus	2 cups / 480 ml	6 g protein
Spinach	2 cups / 480 ml	2 g protein
Kale	2 cups / 480 ml	4 g protein
Swiss chard	2 cups / 480 ml	2 g protein
Bean sprouts	2 cups / 480 ml	2 g protein
Oatmeal	1 cup / 240 ml	6 g protein
Quinoa	1 cup / 240 ml prepared	8 g protein
Edamame	1 cup / 240 ml prepared	17 g protein
Tempeh	1 cup / 240 ml	31 g protein
Tofu	5 oz / 142 g	10 g protein
Hemp Protein Powder (1 scoop)	30 g	15.5 g protein
Rice Protein Powder (1 scoop)	30 g	12 g protein
Whey Protein Powder (1 scoop)	30 g	27 g protein
Soy Protein Powder (1 scoop)	30 g	25 g protein

acceptable as a protein source when following the *Eat-Clean Diet Stripped* plan. That does not mean all soy products are okay, however. Soy has crept its way into a seemingly endless array of foods. It's used to replace meat in foods that are vegetarian but definitely not Clean, and it's used in very unhealthy prepared food. Make sure you read the ingredients of any soy product you're thinking of consuming.

Tempeh is an ideal soy-based food and is made by fermenting whole soybeans. This process increases the vitamin, mineral and protein content of soy. The fermentation process also results in increased bioavailability of the protein in soy. Tempeh is normally cut into slices or cubes and then marinated before cooking.

Some controversy exists around the consumption of soy products. Some studies suggest soy helps prevent cancer where others show it may contribute to causing cancer. Soy has been demonstrated to help prevent heart disease. Some people are concerned about its phytoestrogens, but research does not support these concerns. Soybeans do provide excellent nutrition and are an important addition to our diet, particularly for those looking to eat less meat. As with most things, moderation is the key. I stick to one or two servings a week.

Protein Powder

Plenty of protein powders contain chemicals, sugar, artificial sugars and a host of other ingredients you don't want in your body, but plenty more are natural. These are extremely useful for anyone who follows the Eat-Clean Diet lifestyle, because adding a scoop of powder to your oats or blending some up for a quick shake is a simple way to get your necessary protein.

> "Soybeans do provide excellent nutrition and are an important addition to our diet."

A BIG CAUTION ON PROTEIN POWDER

As I repeat constantly about everything you put in your mouth, read the ingredients! Tons of protein-powder manufacturers add sweeteners, artificial sweeteners, colors and flavors along with other chemicals. Just because you buy it at the same place you buy your all-natural foods and supplements does not mean the protein is natural.

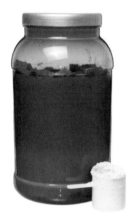

▲ OPT FOR UNSWEETENED protein powders or those that are naturally flavored.

Protein powders are the ultimate in convenience, especially for vegetarians. Choose from rice, soy, pea and hemp or create your own using flaxseed and chia seed. You can add protein to practically any dish, but most protein powders can only be cooked up to 350°F / 177°C, so be cautious when cooking with these powders.

Protein is a great addition to your morning oatmeal and it promotes muscle repair when added to a post-workout shake.

Gluten-Free Eating

In recent years countless people have begun eating gluten free. For some this is a necessity, as they either have celiac disease, a gluten intolerance or a wheat allergy. For others it is a choice because they feel their bodies simply function better without gluten. Whatever your reasons for keeping a gluten-free diet, the *Eat-Clean Diet Stripped* program is for you! There is no easier program for eating gluten free than this one.

The ease with which you move into a gluten-free *Stripped* diet depends very much on what you're used to eating. If you're in the habit of eating pre-packaged convenience foods or sandwiches for many of your meals, you will find it far more difficult than if you are already in the habit of Eating Clean, but happen to have a few extra pounds clinging to your waistline.

People who have the hardest time adapting to a gluten-free life in general are those whose diets normally consist of breads, muffins and other flour-based items, along with packaged foods. When you Eat Clean, these items are not a major part of your diet if they are a part of your diet at all. Think about the way food grows and how it is harvested, and then eat it as close to that way as possible.

Following the *Stripped* program while staying gluten free could not be easier. Most gluten-containing foods are either not a part of this plan at all or it's easy to opt not to eat them. The majority of the *Stripped* plan is made up of lean proteins and vegetables. These are all gluten free, and this program does not allow for possibly gluten-containing sauces and dips.

Grains and starchy carbohydrates are allowed in limited amounts, but it's easy to make sure these are gluten free. Opt for quinoa and you've got a high-protein, gluten-free grain. Who needs wheat? Uncontaminated oats are also gluten free. You'll have a little more trouble once you have lost your final 10 and are maintaining your weight, but the concept is the same. Keep a diet that consists of lean proteins, vegetables and fruit, all in their most natural state.

Often when people find they have intolerance to a food, they concentrate on the items they can no longer eat. I urge you instead to look at the items you can eat – the list is practically endless! The following is a list of gluten-free foods. This list is by no means exhaustive; there are plenty more options. But I have no doubt that in looking at this list you will be inspired to create any number of delicious gluten-free meals.

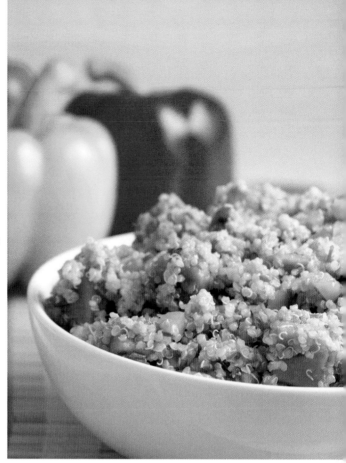

▲ **QUINOA SALAD,** containing fresh vegetables and herbs, is the perfect vegetarian Eat-Clean meal.

"There is no easier program for eating gluten free than this one."

Gluten-Free Foods

OFTEN WHEN WE DISCOVER we have a food intolerance or allergy we moan about all the foods we can no longer have. I like to have a more positive approach, so here is a list of all the foods you can have when you're both gluten free and stripping off those last 10!

Grains:

Uncontaminated oats

Quinoa

Brown rice

Produce:

Apples

Bananas

Plums

Lemons

Blueberries

Raspberries

Strawberries

Pears

Tomatoes

Cucumber

Broccoli

Asparagus

Carrots

Beets

Leeks

Spinach

Sweet potatoes

Brussels sprouts

Green beans

Onions

Radishes

Sprouts

Romaine lettuce

Celery

Dairy:

Eggs

Almond milk

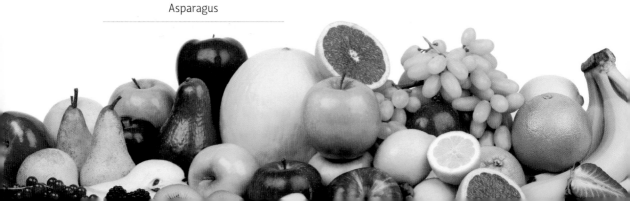

Protein:

Chicken breast

Turkey breast

Trout

Bison

Tilapia

Canned tuna, water-packed

Soy / Edamame

Nuts/Seeds:

Walnuts

Flaxseed

Almonds

Cashews

Oils/Condiments:

Hummus

Almond butter

Miscellaneous

Gluten-free protein powder

Cinnamon

You may notice that this list is exactly the same as the list for people who are not gluten free. Yes, really! Once you begin to maintain your weight on *The Eat-Clean Diet* "Cooler 2" plan (see page 154), you will have even more selection. Once you go Clean, gluten free is simple.

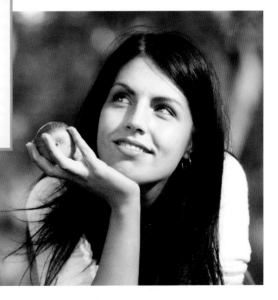

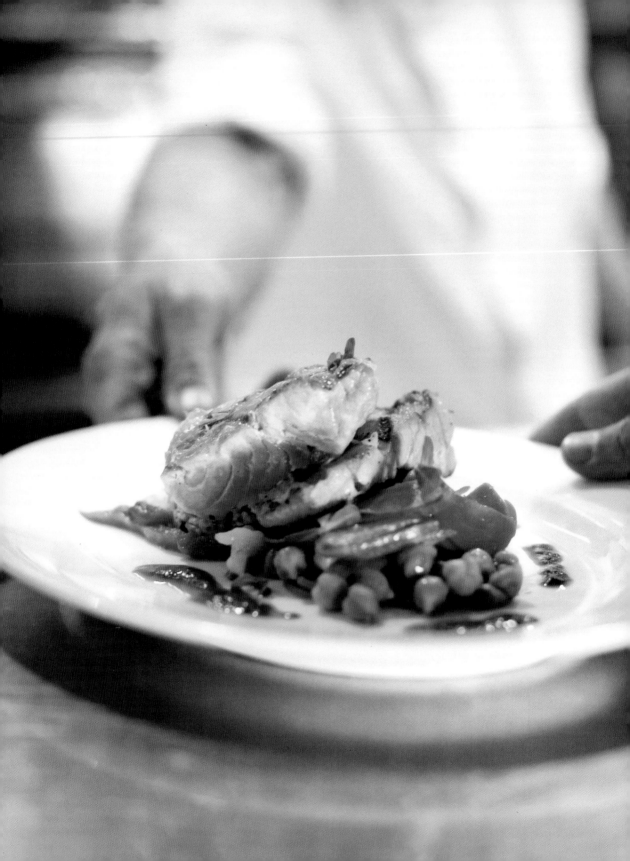

7 Eating Out – Restaurants, Coffee Shops and Social Events

At this moment I am sitting on a plane thousands of feet up in the sky. Planes are generally not known for their nutritious fare, a fact I am keenly aware of thanks to the countless trips I have made up there. Just thinking about what I might face on that rickety airplane cart gives me a sick feeling in my stomach, enough to make me do everything possible to avoid "it" – "it" being the rustling packets of junk food, stale cookies, squished sandwiches, greasy pizza and so on.

I have come to expect lame food offerings on the road, so I take responsibility for my nutrition by packing a few staple items in my carry-on luggage. I'm not talking full hot meals, but I do pack a few dry goods to serve in an emergency. This normally means several small plastic zipper bags into which I have measured about a third of a cup of dry oats, two tablespoons of ground flaxseed, one tablespoon of wheat germ and one scoop of protein powder. The packets store well and provide me, in the presence of hot water, with a nourishing meal that will appease my hunger for a while. I also pack some tea bags, and I'm all set!

In this fast-paced world almost everyone is on the road or in the air, yet most of us do not plan adequately for hunger while we're out there. It's odd, because eating is something we humans do quite a lot. Unprepared we are much more likely to sidle up to a drive-thru speaker. When you are desperate to eat, nothing can stop you from munching everything in sight. Planning is one of the best solutions to this scenario.

When you are eating out, you need a game plan. You should avoid eating out as much as possible while following the *Eat-Clean Diet Stripped* plan because once you enter a restaurant, you

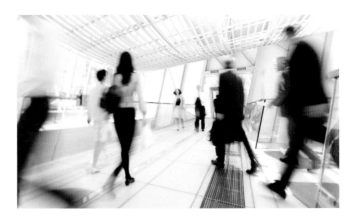

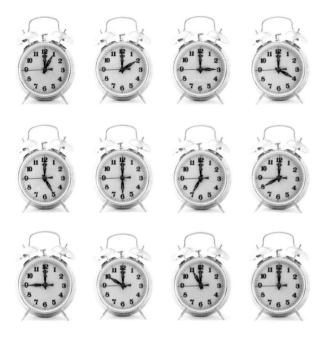

"When you are desperate to eat, nothing can stop you from munching everything in sight. Planning is one of the best solutions to this scenario."

surrender control over what is in your food. That being said, in reality you will likely find yourself at a restaurant during these 28 days.

Many of these situations come as part of your job. For example, as I write this I am on my way to Atlanta to attend a fitness show where I will be judging a contest and conducting an Eat-Clean seminar tomorrow. My day begins at 7:00 AM when I will be hosting a breakfast. Then I move on to judging for four hours. I will take a small break and move on to hosting my seminar, and from there I move into more judging which will end around midnight, but could run much longer depending on how organized the show is. Nowhere in the schedule is there a time given to eat. I realize I will have to depend on what food may be available at the host hotel, and on what I have prepared for myself and could bring along on the trip.

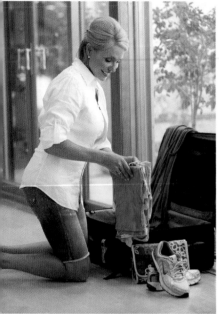

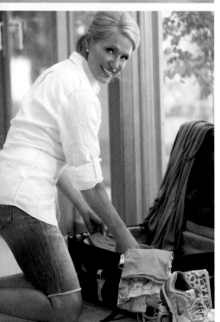

Flying from Canada to the United States does not allow for many food options. Fruit and vegetables are verboten! So when I arrive in Atlanta I will head off to a nearby grocery store to fill my cooler with Clean food. This I will bring to the event and carry with me all day. At the hotel I will request only Clean options. Since this is a work event I already know I won't be drinking alcohol – I rarely do anyway, and especially not when I'm trying to drop a few pounds.

I want you to learn how to prepare yourself for eating out, in case you must. There are several easy strategies that will help you sort out what works and what doesn't for your *Stripped* eating plan. Here are my top 10 eating-out strategies to help make you leaner at the end of the day.

Top 10 Eating-Clean / Eating-Out Strategies

① Develop an "I Don't Have To Eat It All!" Mindset.

Make up your mind before you go that it does not have to be a most-bang-for-your-buck experience. Many people become a little unhinged when they see a menu exploding with delicious options. Keep your goal in mind.

② Satisfy Hunger Only – Don't Gorge.

Eat for the purpose of satisfying your hunger, but no more. The point of eating is to refuel your body at various intervals throughout the day with just enough nourishment to accomplish that task. Food supplies the raw materials used to repair, rebuild, grow and maintain your body. Eat just enough to feel satisfied but not stuffed.

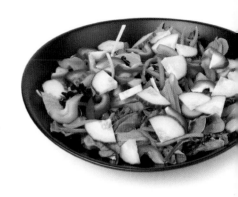

③ Start Small and Green.
Start your meal with a salad, without dressing. Use a spritz of lemon or some balsamic vinegar. Choosing a salad will give you another opportunity to load up on fibrous foods that fill up your stomach.

④ Broth is Best.
When there is no Clean salad option, have a broth-based soup. Ask your server whether the soup contains cream, and if so then skip the soup. You may also have to request no extra dollops such as sour cream. These too are often high in fats and calories, more unwanted intruders in your *Stripped* plan.

⑤ No Bread, Please.
Forgo the breadbasket. Your salad will be arriving shortly. If you really can't resist the bread offerings, be sure to choose a whole-grain variety, drizzle on some heart-healthy olive oil rather than butter and stick to one piece only. Remember, this is not helping you reach your 10-pound weight-loss goal.

⑥ Clean Cooking Techniques Rock!
Look for entrée options featuring steamed or raw vegetables and grilled, baked or roasted meats or fish. If these options aren't there, ask for them anyway. You can't go wrong with a grilled chicken breast and steamed vegetables, no butter or sauce. And don't go by "low fat" or "heart healthy" symbols. Studies show these choices are often not as they appear.

⑦ Portion Control Is In.
Have a good look at your plate when your food arrives. How big is the plate and how much food is on it? North Americans have grown so accustomed to super-sized portions that we

"You can't go wrong with a grilled chicken breast and steamed vegetables, no butter or sauce."

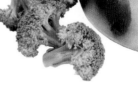

don't recognize what is too much. Request a doggie bag right away if the portion is larger than we suggest on page 64. Take half home or back to the hotel and have it the next day.

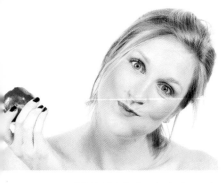

▲ **TAKE THE TIME** to slowly chew and really taste the food you're eating – it is meant to be enjoyed.

⑧ Fletcherize.

Fletcherizing is the practice of chewing each mouthful of food a minimum of 25 times. Doing this gives your body time to recognize that you are slowly becoming full and satiated. If we gobble our food (I was a gobbler in my past life), we tend to eat more. Aim to take at least 20 minutes to eat your food. This much chewing also pre-digests your food in your mouth, helps release more nutrients and helps prevent gas.

⑨ Zero Tolerance.

Every time I give an *Eat-Clean Diet* seminar the question of alcohol comes up, because it is so much a part of our social behavior. It will do us good to remember that alcohol is made from sugar. You will want to avoid alcohol during your *Stripped* plan because sugar will derail you in a most powerful way. To stay hydrated and to fill your empty hand, have sparkling or regular water with slices of fresh lemon or lime.

⑩ Stop Before the End.

Though temptation may arrive on a dessert tray at the end of your meal, this is not the time to succumb. Think of your plan to shed those irritating 10 final pounds and redouble your efforts by reaching for a decaf black coffee instead. Can't do it? Ask for a small bowl of fresh fruit and leave it at that. You can't build a lean, tight body on the back of sweets and temptation.

Three More Helpful Tips

① Pre-Eat.

If you doubt your ability to resist restaurant offerings, try a little trick called "pre-eating." I will eat a Clean meal before meeting business associates or friends. Then when I am at the restaurant or social event, I don't have to worry about being hungry or eating foods that don't bring me to my goals. I order a water or a coffee and focus on conversation.

② Make Nice with the Wait Staff.

Be friendly with your server. You may have to request some special food prepared and you want your server on your side. You can request that items such as cheese, gravy, sauces, dressings, butter and fries not be served with your entrée. Be prepared to send the food back politely if it appears with an unwanted item on it.

③ Eat Clean at the Drive Thru.

Familiarize yourself with the menu of any fast-food drive-thru establishments. I don't frequent such places much myself, but I do know that you can Eat Clean there if you prepare. Portions at fast-food places are already enormous, so never super size what you purchase unless you plan on sharing. Make smart food choices by ordering grilled chicken, fish or turkey-based menu items. The more sauce- and dressing-free greens and veggies you can squeeze into your meal, the better it is for your *Stripped* plan. Avoid obvious no-nos such as milkshakes, fries and other greasy, fried offerings. These have no place in your *Stripped* plan. If you are eating these foods, you are not serious about losing weight.

"Avoid obvious no-nos such as milkshakes, fries and other greasy, fried offerings. These have no place in your *Stripped* plan. If you are eating these foods, you are not serious about losing weight."

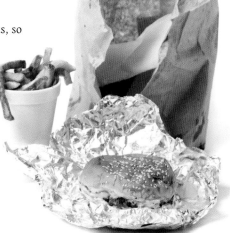

Make Your Friendships Your Focus!

ONE OF THE MOST DIFFICULT THINGS to manage while following a healthy lifestyle plan is your social life. So much of the time we spend with friends and family is tied to drinking alcohol and eating, two things that you must adjust if you're going to lose those last 10 pounds! Fear not, here's a list of things you can do with your friends and family that will not compromise your fitness goals!

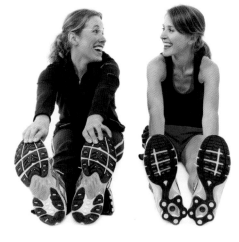

(1) GYM PARTNERS. This is an obvious one! Is there any better place to have a friend than at the gym? Working out together allows friends to do what they do best: support each other.

(2) GAMES NIGHT. Instead of going out for dinner, invite the girls in for a night of board-game fun! You provide the Clean snacks and they'll provide you a night filled with laughs!

(3) BATTERS UP. There are many adult sports leagues that range from beginner to advanced. Form a team with your friends and you can play any sport from basketball to softball to dodgeball all year long! You'll also open yourself to meeting other people who are just as interested in being fit as you are!

(4) GET CREATIVE. Take a photography class or learn to make pottery, sculpt, knit or paint. After the class, you can collaborate on projects and spend time being creative together.

(5) VOLUNTEER TOGETHER. Make time with your friends really count by volunteering your time to a charity. Find something everyone is passionate about and convert your social time into social capital.

(6) EXPERIENCE CULTURE. Visit your town's museums, galleries and festivals. Together with your friends you can experience art, music and the culture of your very own city. Many cities have their own websites where these events are posted. Pick a new place each week, gather up your girls and get ready to talk about all of the wonderful things you've seen that day.

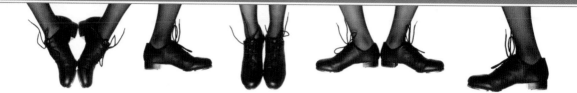

7 JUST DANCE. With the popularity of reality television dance shows, I know many people who have taken up dancing classes of all kinds. Many studios offer adult belly dancing, ballroom, hip-hop, tap and even ballet dancing. These classes offer you and your friends the chance to hang out together while having fun!

Of course there are times when you'll end up at dinner with friends and you should enjoy yourself! I usually check the menus for restaurants online beforehand and look for a healthy option. If there isn't anything that fits the Eat-Clean Principles, I eat my Clean meal before dinner so I'm not tempted at the restaurant. Once I'm with my friends, I get lost in all the conversation anyway!

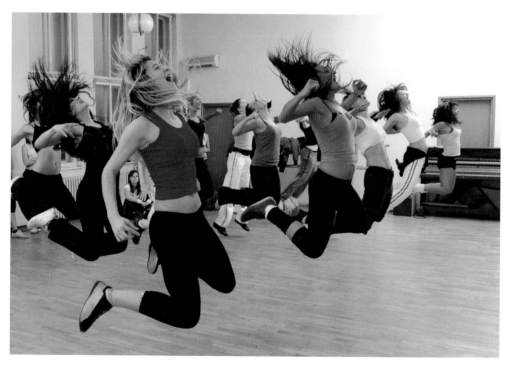

▲ **DANCE CLASSES** such as Zumba, hip-hop cardio and ballet don't seem like workouts because they're so much fun!

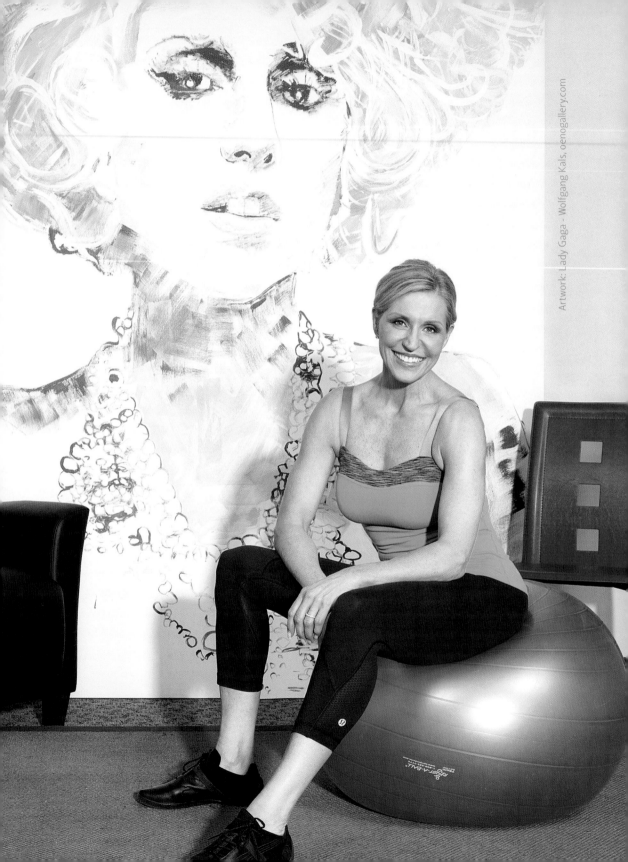

8 | Your Stripped-Down Workout Routine

IN ancient times athletes wore nothing at all. Their physiques showed exactly who they were and what they did. At the esteemed Louvre in Paris, France, you can see a spear thrower's chiseled arms and torso bursting with power, and a discus thrower putting his entire unclothed body into his effort. Ancient athletes were proud citizens who worked hard for their distinction. Not only did their bodies show beautifully, they were regarded as special people who contributed to their society.

> "Walking should be part of your basic effort to become more mobile, as it will help you shed those unwanted final pounds."

Today we offer our skills to our community in different ways – most often not with a naked, ripped physique. Goodness knows it is difficult to become an elite athlete, but earning a decent physique bearing little fat and showing lean muscle is within grasp. Spending seven days on your feet touring a legendary city like Paris, for example, can help you shed weight – particularly if you follow up with Clean food. Yes, even in Paris this is possible. How many Clean meals did I eat while I recently vacationed there? With the exception of a few celebratory occasions, my meals were based on haricots verts, poulet et riz brun. Remarkably the walking helped me keep my body in line throughout my visit. I went down an entire dress size during that time!

Walking is the most basic movement you can do with your body after getting up off the couch. Nothing is required except lacing up your sneakers. You just place one foot in front of the other. Incidentally it may interest you to know that when you join a running group to prepare for your first 5k, you will be instructed to walk/run until you work your way up in running ability. Walking should be part of your basic effort to become more mobile, as it will help you shed those unwanted final pounds.

Take advantage of every opportunity to walk more each day. Walk to work. Walk to the grocery store. Walk to pick up the cleaning. Walk to school. Walk the dog. Go for a walk with your family. Walk, walk, walk and then walk some more. We should not embrace the notion of using wheels to get around unless those wheels are attached to a bicycle and we are pedaling. I see a worrisome trend of folks reaching for some format of wheeled transportation – segways, cars and so on – when they could easily use their own feet to do the same job. I am not talking about people for whom a wheelchair is necessary. Healthy folks need to walk more. Start today. It doesn't cost a dime and it feels sweet to be on your feet.

Once your shoes are on, you simply need to think of good reasons to become a pedestrian. You can get anywhere if you are willing to give your feet a nudge out the door. When I go on vacation, no matter where the city, I lose weight because I am moving all day long. I mentioned Paris. The same was true on previous vacations to Barcelona in Spain and Rangiroa in the South Pacific. Heck, if you need to book a vacation to lose weight, then do it!

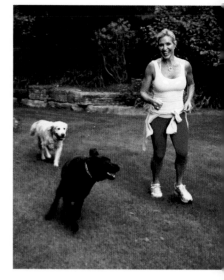

▲ **SPENDING TIME ON YOUR FEET,** especially outdoors, is good for both your body and your mind.

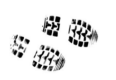 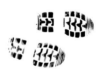 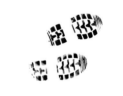

The ancient Greeks used good, hard physical endeavors to hone a body. They may not have had weights as we know them today, but if you combine the efforts of weight training with cardiovascular work and eat a Clean diet, you will create hard muscle to replace the layer of fat. Never lifted a weight? Don't worry. Weight training is for everyone. Keep in mind that I was a complete novice with regard to weight training before I overhauled my own physique. Today you can't peel me away from the weight rack. Training with weights is my salvation.

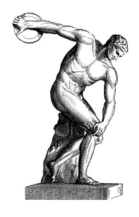

How do you get the same kind of passion for something that looks so intimidating? You will need to have patience with yourself. Acquiring new skills takes time. Your first time doing anything you are likely to feel awkward and a little foolish. This should not keep you from trying again, perfecting your technique and being willing to look a little foolish on occasion. As with every new endeavor you need to do it 10 times before it becomes a habit. Give yourself at least that much time.

It's okay to feel intimidated about hoisting a weight over your head. Everyone feels that way the first time holding iron dumbbells. It's out of the norm. Never mind; with dedication and a plan the time will come when you will be firm, strong and confident lifting weights. Don't give up. Keep your eye on the plan you have crafted for yourself and make it happen.

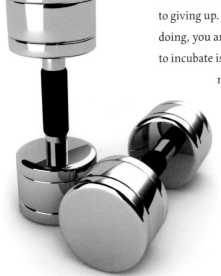

▼ **WEIGHTS MAY LOOK** intimidating, but they are really just conveniently shaped heavy objects.

In my early days of weight training I leaned heavily on friends who were also interested in the sport. I needed their help and their enthusiasm. That got me through times when I was close to giving up. Research also shows that what your friends are doing, you are doing, so finding friends with the habit you want to incubate is a great idea. I also always carried a copy of *Oxygen* magazine in my gym bag, because I wanted to review how to do the exercises before my workout. All training articles became mandatory reading for me! A personal trainer can help you with motivation. This is what they are paid to do. Personal trainers will come to your home or will do the job at a gym, whichever you prefer.

Basic Training Routine For the Novice

CARDIOVASCULAR ACTIVITY:

You will need to schedule at least three cardiovascular sessions per week. Every other day should include some sort of activity that will get your heart rate up and keep it there for a good 30 minutes or more. You can keep track of your heart rate using a heart rate monitor or you can try the talk test. Runnersworld.com explains the talk test as an inexpensive but effective way of measuring how much you are exerting yourself by whether or not you can still talk comfortably as you run. This ensures that you are not exerting your heart and lungs too much. Exercising above this intensity level pushes you out of your aerobic-conditioning zone (the aerobic exercise level that produces maximum long-term training effects), and it becomes hard to sustain exercise for any length of time.

You will also want to be aware, particularly because you are a beginner, that your heart and lungs work at various intensities. The Lance Armstrongs of the world are so finely tuned physically that their heart and lungs work well even when they push themselves as hard as they possibly can, but most of us will never be at that point. The ideal level of exertion you need to reach during cardiovascular exercise is one where optimal fat burning takes place. Plenty of studies show that being active at 50 to 60 percent of your maximum heart rate (MHR), three times per week for at least 30 minutes each time will maintain heart health, but to blast fat you will need to train at a level higher than 60 percent of your MHR. Once you have achieved an intermediate level of fitness and want to get even leaner, train at 70 to 80 percent of your MHR, a rate that promotes aerobic conditioning as well as weight loss.

YOUR BEGINNER EXERCISE NEEDS

First undergo a complete medical check up to assess you are well enough to begin an exercise program.

Have on hand:

→ **Water bottle(s)**

→ **Small towel**

→ **Comfortable clothing**

→ **Proper gym shoes**

→ **Training journal**

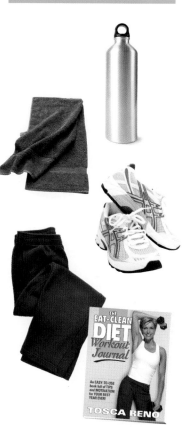

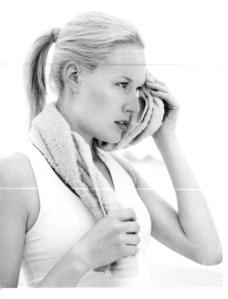

Weight training is critical not only for keeping you toned and tight, but also for improving bone density, maintaining daily living activities such as picking up those heavy grocery bags laden with Clean eats, and increasing your basic metabolism, helping you burn energy even at rest.

Many beginners are afraid weight training will leave them looking like Arnold Schwarzenegger's body double. I guarantee this won't happen unless you are genetically inclined to be that way and you consciously try to accomplish this feat. I would like you to think of weight training as a way of creating a physique that is strong and healthy, with beauty as an added bonus.

Walking into a gym can be overwhelming for the beginner. My own first experience left me timid and very unsure of my abilities. *Oxygen* magazine in hand, I walked into my local gym with my hat pulled down and my headphones in. This training time was all about *me* and building *my* physique, and I didn't allow myself to worry about the other people there.

I found great benefit from working with personal trainers. They introduced me to fitness equipment and taught me the ins and outs of the weight room. I wasn't intimidated by the buff men grunting in the weight pen once I knew how to use the weights and had my own plan of attack. Keep your own goals in mind when you hit the gym. Post your efforts and your ever-changing goals in your training journal to motivate you each time you train. Still uncomfortable? You can outfit your home with exercise equipment to begin your training there.

DEVELOPING YOUR TRAINING PLAN

Overload:
Your muscles need to be challenged with each repetition in order to build strength. On your last repetition you should have to work hard to finish without losing your form.

Progression:
Your body is a smart, efficient machine. Over time you will need to change your plan in order to continually challenge it. You can do so by increasing your repetitions, then increasing your weight and/or changing exercises for that particular muscle. In general you should switch up your weight lifting routine every three to five weeks.

We have prepared an effective yet simple training plan to work with your *Stripped* nutrition plan. Please take a look on page 124 for a gym workout followed by a home workout. You can make the following adjustments to make starting easier for you:

→ Start with very low weights or no weights at all.

→ Start with one set instead of two or three.

→ Start with high repetitions within the 15 to 20 range instead of 12 to 15.

→ Focus on your breathing, exhaling with each contraction and inhaling with each relaxation.

→ Take one-minute breaks after finishing one exercise before starting another.

→ Pay special attention to your posture and technique when lifting weights to avoid injury.

→ Do the plan twice a week until you feel comfortable enough with the exercises to move up to three times each week.

→ Warm up your body for five minutes before your workout by walking on the spot, on the treadmill or stepping up on stairs or a bench.

→ Cool down adequately with a total body stretch session.

Initially you may feel stiffness in your muscles after your first few sessions. Don't let this scare you off. This stiffness means the exercise is working! You will soon interpret this feeling as good pain. If the pain is more than you can manage, perhaps you started a little too gung-ho. Just reduce the weight slightly. Remember to give each muscle 24 to 48 hours' recovery time before training it again, to decrease your chances of overtraining and give your body a chance to do what the workout was meant to – build muscle tissue! Overall, weight training will work wonders for your body but it will take a few sessions to adjust to the routine. You're a Sister in Iron once you've lifted your first weight. Join us in the crusade as we pump iron one rep at a time.

"You're a Sister in Iron once you've lifted your first weight. Join us in the crusade as we pump iron one rep at a time."

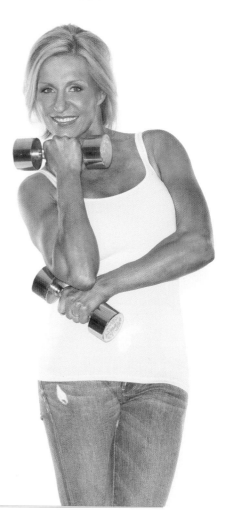

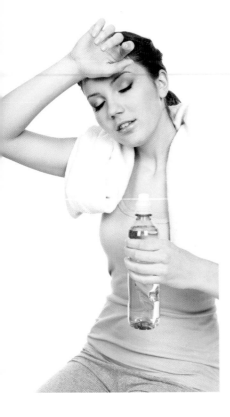

The Workout

Exercise and Eating Clean go hand in hand. While maintaining your diet will bring you 80 percent of the distance, according to the Body Beautiful/Body Healthy 80-10-10 formula on page 15, you won't get the *Stripped* body you're looking for unless you exercise as well. I have worked out a no-nonsense plan to keep you burning fat all day long.

During your 28-day *Stripped* plan you'll be eating differently than you are currently accustomed to. Your food will be of a higher nutritional value and therefore more nourishing and satisfying, but you may crave certain foods you are used to having. If you are already in the habit of working out hard, you may have to modify your workouts so as not to put your body too far into a state of depletion. The goal is to feel great, have abundant energy and to strip excess pounds from your body. After the 28-day plan has ended and you have achieved your 10-pound loss, it's important to revamp your plan to incorporate more vigorous exercise. This is vital to help you succeed long term as you increase your food consumption on your maintenance plan (see page 154).

"If you are already in the habit of working out hard, you may have to modify your workouts so as not to put your body too far into a state of depletion."

A critical aspect of your training is the tracking of your progress. People who set goals and track their progress are twice as likely to achieve success as those who don't. An interesting experiment reveals this likelihood. Scientists conducted experiments on students writing exams. Half of the class was told to go ahead and write their exams. They were given no special instructions. Before the other half wrote their exams they were told to record the mark they hoped to get at the top right hand of the paper. When students did this they always performed better. In other words, they set themselves up for success before they had started! This is what I want you to do – place success firmly at the top of your mind right from the start. You can use a simple notebook or a journal such as *The Eat-Clean Diet Workout Journal* to help you during these four exciting weeks and long after you've reached your goals, too.

The following plan has been created for intermediate to advanced exercisers. If you are a beginner, please refer to page 117 for your beginner modifications.

Your *Stripped* Weight-Loss Exercise Plan

Sunday	Monday	Tuesday	Wednesday	Thursday	Friday	Saturday
Rest Day	Weights	Endurance Cardio	Weights	Interval Training Cardio	Weights	Endurance Cardio

Cardiovascular Training

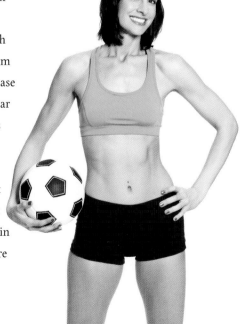

Cardiovascular training is extremely important for the efficiency and health of your heart and circulatory system, as well as your metabolism. Your heart is a powerful muscle that endlessly pumps nutrients and oxygen to, and waste products from, each and every cell in your body. In order to condition it for optimum function you need to utilize other large muscle groups to increase the flow of blood throughout your body. The best cardiovascular activity is the kind you love, and can do for at least 30 minutes at a go. I love to swim, cycle, run, dive and play soccer. My daughters love to dance. Others like to play organized sports, golf or belly dance. Whatever you do, be sure to choose a sport or activity you will enjoy so you will stick to it. Don't overlook the simplest activity of all – walking! Simply putting one foot in front of the other can be quite demanding, depending on where and at what intensity you do it.

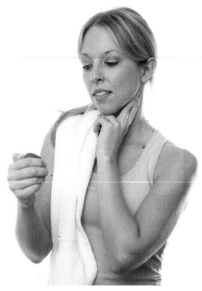

For successful cardiovascular training you should become familiar with your heart rate. Each of us is programmed with a maximum heart rate. Some of us operate at a higher heart rate than others. We are all different. When exercising, your heart rate in comparison to your maximum will determine which type of training you are doing. Here's a simple way to calculate your maximum heart rate:

Calculate Your Maximum Heart Rate (MHR):

Formula: 220 - age = Maximum Heart Rate

Example for a 20-year-old: 220 – 20 = 200 beats per minute (bpm)

"A great way to get in shape quickly is to alternate between low-intensity and high-intensity training."

A great way to get in shape quickly is to alternate between low-intensity and high-intensity training. A low-intensity plan makes your heart work at 60 to 70 percent of your MHR. For example, when running you wouldn't be sprinting at your fastest speed, nor would you be ambling. Instead you would run at a moderate pace that will challenge your heart but not leave you breathless or feeling like you are going to throw up. You will perform two sessions of low-intensity aerobic cardiovascular exercise each week, working within your individual heart-rate range, for 30 to 40 minutes per session.

Example of a Moderate-Intensity Heart Rate Range:

220 – 20 = 200 bpm x 0.6 = 120 bpm

220 – 20 = 200 bpm x 0.7 = 140 bpm

If you are 20 years old, your moderate-intensity heart rate range is between 120 and 140 bpm.

Understanding Fuel Consumption

Nope, I'm not talking about your car! Here's a brief science lesson on your body's consumption of fuel during exercise. The three systems required for creating energy your muscles can use during exercise are glycolysis, the Krebs cycle (or citric acid cycle) and the electron transport chain. These three fancy systems are fine tuned to produce energy based on oxygen levels.

Glucose (sugar) is the body's main fuel source. When it is burned to release fuel for the muscles, the end product is an important chemical called pyruvate. In the presence of oxygen (this is called aerobic exercise), pyruvate will enter the Krebs cycle, which employs fat products and creates lots of energy for your muscles. Without oxygen present (this is called anaerobic exercise) the pyruvate is converted to lactic acid. Lactate builds up in your muscles, creating an uncomfortable burning sensation.

During anaerobic exercise your muscles quickly burn up available glucose, leaving you without enough fuel to keep up the demand on your muscles. You are left feeling fatigued. When you work at a high intensity of aerobic exercise, you are flirting with your anaerobic threshold. Working at this level forces your system to raise your anaerobic threshold, which will enable you to work at a higher intensity while still being able to burn fat as fuel rather than relying solely on glucose. This means you can exercise harder for longer while burning tons of fat!

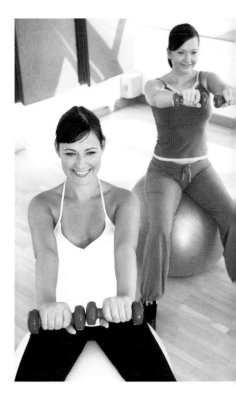

▼ **FEELING THE BURN** after a workout is a good thing, so long as the soreness goes away in a couple of days.

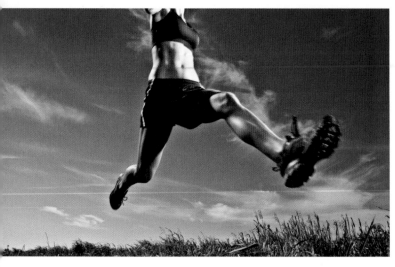

Interval training conditions both your aerobic and anaerobic systems to use energy more efficiently. This is the ultimate in fat burning. You can train in the anaerobic zone for only a short period of time, but training at that intensity burns enormous amounts of calories. By giving yourself an aerobic rest between anaerobic sessions during the same workout, you get the best of both worlds – a longer session than you could do anaerobically, but with huge calorie-burning benefits. I encourage performing at least one session of interval training each week.

Doing HIIT (high-intensity interval training) on the treadmill for 30 minutes will burn far more calories than doing a consistent pace for the same 30 minutes. You will be pouring with sweat by the time you complete your interval training, I promise! High-intensity interval training works like this: perform intervals of high-intensity training alternated with intervals of moderate intensity. It's easy and rapidly produces results, both in calorie burning and improved fitness. Here's how to calculate your high intensity:

> "High-intensity interval training works like this: perform intervals of high-intensity training alternated with intervals of moderate intensity."

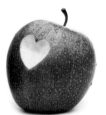

High-Intensity Heart Rate Range:
220 - 20 = 200 bpm x 0.75 = 150 bpm
220 - 20 = 200 bpm x 0.85 = 170 bpm
Your high-intensity heart rate range
is between 150 and 170 bpm.

Your 25-Minute *Stripped* Interval-Training Plan:

Warm Up:

3 minutes – 60 percent maximum heart rate

Intervals (repeat this 14 times):

1 minute – 65 percent

30 seconds – 85 percent

Cool Down:

4 minutes – 60 percent

Weight Training

During your *Stripped* plan it's important to maintain muscle mass, bone density and definition. Most diets encourage weight loss no matter the source. Starving yourself, counting calories or severely restricting food intake usually results in the loss of muscle tissue, which is a disaster for your metabolism. Why? Muscle tissue is the most metabolically active tissue in the body. When you lose it your metabolism drops and you have a harder time burning fat. You will also feel sluggish and tired if you rob your body of muscle. This is definitely not how we strip fat from your body on the *Stripped* program! Regular weight-training sessions will help define your muscles, while cardio and a proper diet will help shed the fat covering up the powerhouse beneath.

I've created a full-body workout routine for you so you can work major muscle groups, burn energy and reveal your sexy, *Stripped*-down muscles in 28 days flat! You will be encouraged by the fact that you will probably see muscular definition in as little as three weeks if you are keeping your diet tight and your training regular. Exciting, isn't it?

"Regular weight-training sessions will help define your muscles, while cardio and a proper diet will help shed the fat covering up the powerhouse beneath."

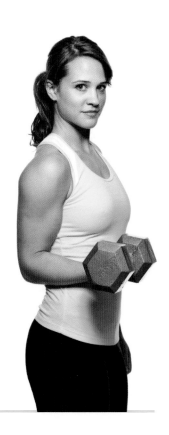

Your *Stripped* Weight-Training Plan

▼ PLAN YOUR WORKOUTS as dates in your schedule. If you want to lose that 10, you'll make the time.

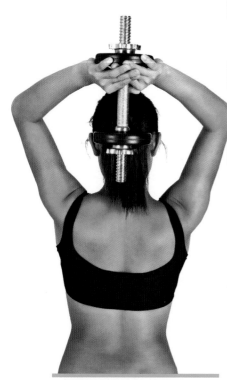

TIP: If you are on a strict budget, check out your local paper or used-goods website for gently used weights and benches for sale. You'll be surprised at how much money you can save this way!

HOW OFTEN?

Three or four times each week.

HOW MANY REPS?

Moderate-high reps: 12 to 15

HOW MANY SETS?

Three sets per exercise.

HOW MUCH WEIGHT?

Use a weight that leaves you genuinely fatigued during the last few repetitions but not so heavy that you lose form.

Training At Home or At the Gym

Just because you want to shed those final 10 pounds doesn't mean you necessarily need to join a gym. Sometimes that is just not in your financial or time budget. Where you train, whether at home or a gym, has little bearing on your end results. It is more important that you do train, and consistently. If you can train at a gym, great – get there now! If you can't, all you need to pull off a fat-burning weight-training workout are a few inexpensive items including a flat bench (adjustable to incline is best) at an average cost of about $150, and several sets of dumbbells varying in weight from five to 25 pounds at $1.50 per pound. Some people like to have a fit ball, which normally costs around $45, but this is not totally necessary. It may be hard to believe, but this is all you will need to build a lean body so there should be nothing standing in your way.

Your *Stripped* Routine at the Gym

Remember to warm up for a few minutes by doing some low-intensity cardio before beginning your weight routine.

Hamstring Curls:

Lie face down on a hamstring-curl bench with the ankle rest adjusted to sit just above your rear ankles. Hold the support handles. Bend your knees until the ankle rest nearly reaches your buttocks. Lower back down with control and repeat.

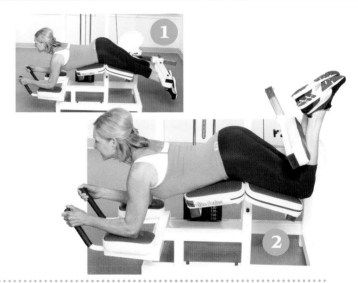

Standing Calf Raises:

Bending slightly, climb under the shoulder pads and lift up to stand straight, your feet hip-width apart. Lower your heels off the edge of the footplate until you feel a slight stretch in your calves. Rise up as high as you can, until you are resting on the balls of your feet. Lower back to the starting position and repeat.

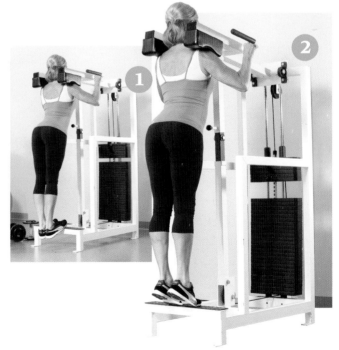

Lat Machine Pulldowns:

Position the seat so your knees are secured under the guard. Hold the bar at a wide grip with even spacing between your hands. Pull the bar down to your sternum while keeping your back tall and flat. Return the bar to the starting position and repeat.

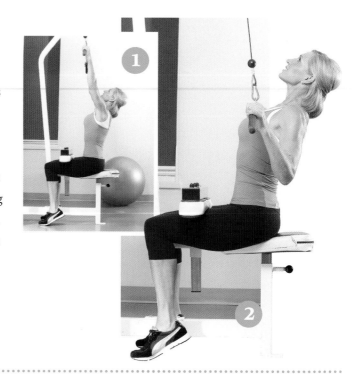

Seated Low Cable Rows:

Sit on the machine's seat or floor with your feet flat on the footrest. Keep a slight bend in your knees. Reach forward and grasp the handle, keeping your back flat. Using your back muscles, pull the handle into your belly. Return to the starting position and repeat.

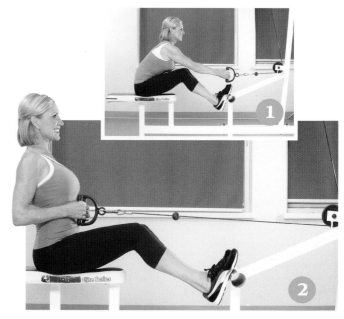

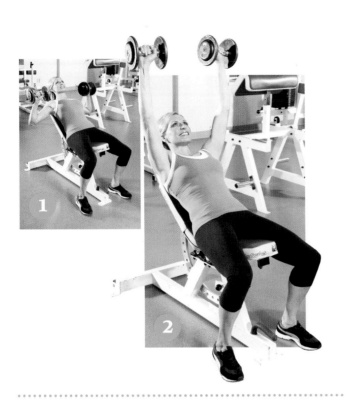
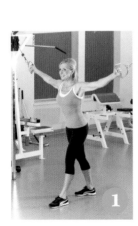
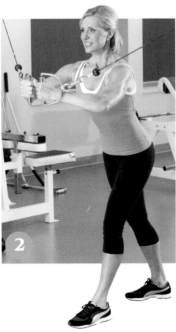

Incline Bench Presses:

Adjust the bench to a 45-degree angle. Lie back on the bench with dumbbells in either hand, held at the outside of your chest. Press the dumbbells out until they meet in front of you by straightening your arms. Return to the starting position and repeat.

Cable Crossovers:

Adjust the cables until your arms are at the desired angle and level. Pull the handles in a hugging-type motion until your hands meet at the middle of your body. If you wish, you can push even further so your hands cross each other at the midpoint. Return to the start position and repeat.

Seated Overhead Shoulder Presses:

Sit on a bench, chair or on the end of a flat bench holding dumbbells in your lap. Lift the dumbbells above your head until your arms are fully extended but not locked. Lower to the shoulders and repeat.

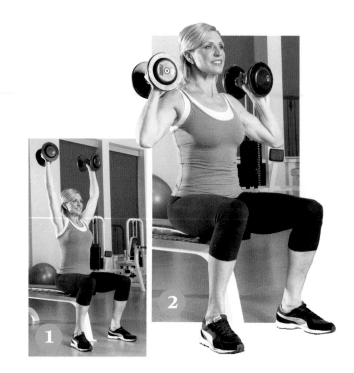

Cable Laterals:

Position the pulley at a level near your feet. Stand next to the pulley machine holding the handle at thigh level in the hand opposite the pulley machine. Pull the handle across your body and up to shoulder height, keeping your arm straight. Complete your repetitions and repeat on the opposite side.

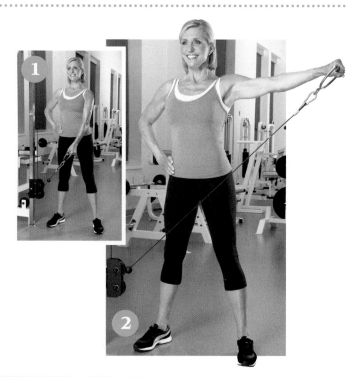

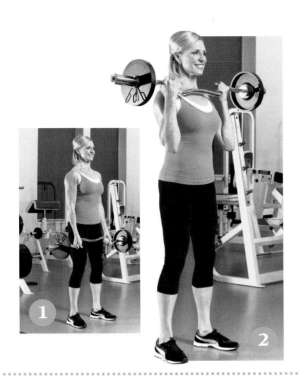

Biceps EZ-Bar Curls:

Either sitting or standing, hold a loaded EZ-bar with a shoulder-width grip. Keeping your elbows at your sides throughout the entire movement, curl the weight up until your arm is completely flexed. Lower back to extension and repeat.

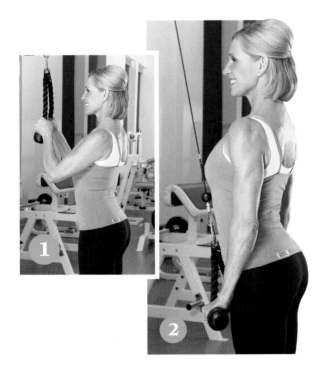

Triceps Rope Pulldowns:

Secure a rope attachment to a cable machine and set the pulley to a high level. Bend your arms, keeping your elbows at your sides. Pull the rope down until your arms are completely extended. Return to the starting position and repeat. Keep your elbows at your sides throughout this movement.

Captain's Chair:

Position yourself on the machine with your back flat against the support and your legs hanging. Using your abdominal muscles, lift your legs. You can lift them straight, as shown, or you can lift your knees to your chest. Lower to the starting position. Repeat.

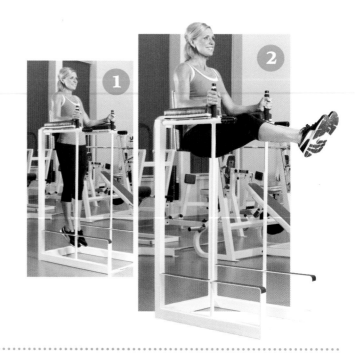

Reverse Crunches:

Lie on a flat bench with your buttocks right at the end. Grasp the upper bench above your head. Using your abdominal muscles, bring your legs up in the air above your hips. Keep a slight bend in your knees and lift your buttocks off the bench in this motion. Lower your legs until your toes nearly touch the floor. Return to starting position, keeping control. Repeat.

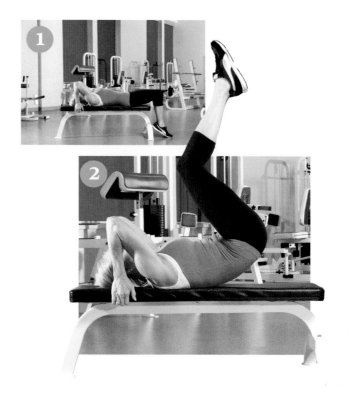

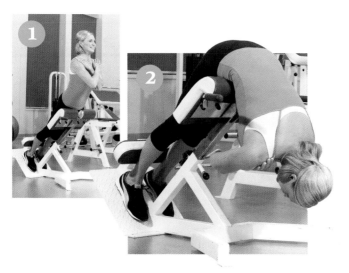

Hyperextensions:

Position the machine until the pads are resting comfortably on your pelvic area. Cross your arms in front of your body or clasp your hands behind your head. Lower your upper body until you are in an inverted V. Use your lower back muscles to return to the starting position. Repeat.

Your *Stripped* Weight-Training Routine at Home

Remember to warm up for a few minutes by doing some low-intensity cardio before beginning your weight routine.

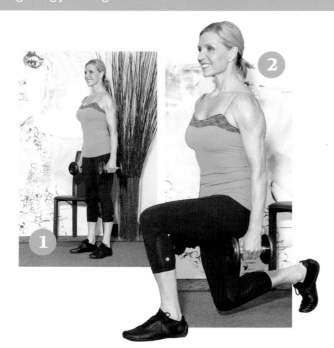

Lunges:

Hold dumbbells in each hand. Step forward with your right leg and bend your knee, keeping it in line with your ankle, until your thigh is parallel to the ground. Make sure your knee does not extend beyond your toe. Keep your back straight. Then return to standing in the forward direction. Repeat movement with the left leg. Alternate legs until the end of the set.

Squats:

Hold a dumbbell in each hand, at shoulder level or with arms straight at your sides. You can also hold a barbell across your shoulders, resting on your trapezius muscle. Place your feet slightly wider than hip-width apart. Keeping your knees in line with your ankles and your back straight, lower your body as if you were sitting in a chair until your thighs are parallel to the ground. Push up to the starting position and repeat.

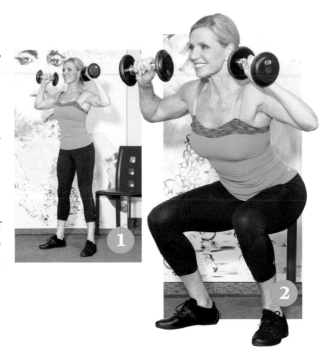

Stiff-Leg Deadlifts:

Hold dumbbells in each hand in front of each thigh. Place your feet hip-width apart. Looking straight ahead and keeping your back flat, lower your upper body until you feel a stretch along the back of your legs. Keep a very slight bend in your knees. Allow your arms to simply hang during this movement. Lift your body until you are standing straight. Repeat.

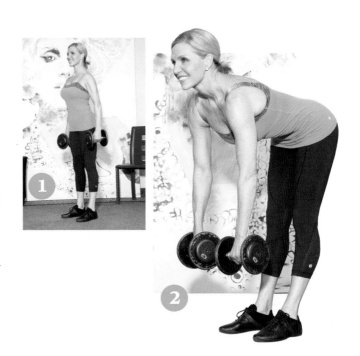

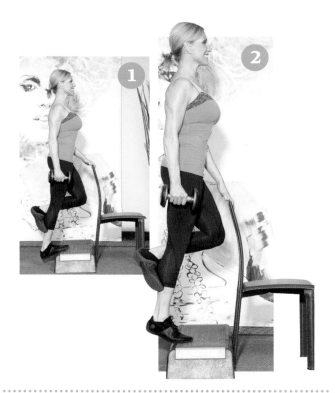

One-Leg Calf Raises on a Step:

Stand on a step or sturdy box. Hold a dumbbell in your left hand and rest your right hand against a chair back, banister or wall for support. Tuck your right foot behind your left ankle. Lower your left heel off the edge of the step until you feel a slight stretch in your calf. Rise up until you are resting on the ball of your foot. Lower the heel back down and repeat. Complete set with one foot, then switch dumbbell to the other hand and repeat with opposite foot.

Bent-Over Rows:

Place your feet slightly wider than hip-width apart. Squat down and pick up your barbell or dumbbells, keeping your back straight. Stand up and bend your knees slightly. Bend forward, keeping your back flat. Pull the weights into your belly at the level of your navel. It helps to focus on a spot across the room at eye level. Return to the starting position and repeat.

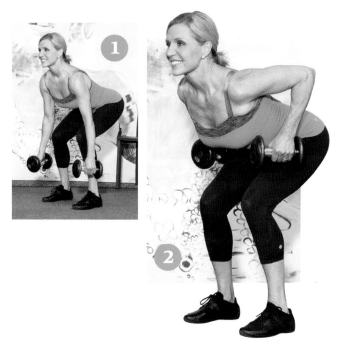

Push Ups:

Place your body into a plank position with your feet together and your legs straight, your extended arms supporting you with your hands under your shoulders. Create a straight line from head to toe. Lower your body to the ground, maintaining a straight line. Push up to the starting position and repeat. If this move is too difficult for you, do a half push up by resting your weight on your knees rather than your toes.

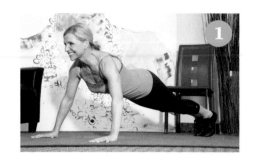

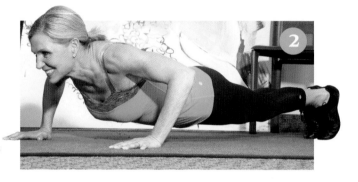

Lateral Raises:

Place a dumbbell in each hand. Stand with your feet hip-width apart and knees slightly bent. You can also sit on a bench or chair for this exercise. Lift your arms straight out to the sides until they reach shoulder height. Keep a "pouring from a pitcher" tilt to your hands, as shown. Return to the starting position and repeat.

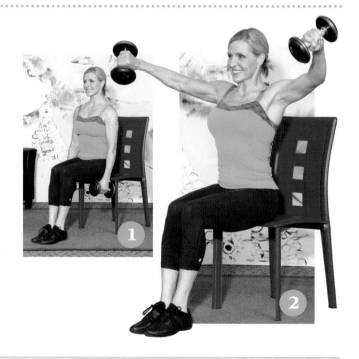

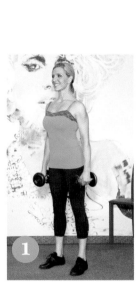

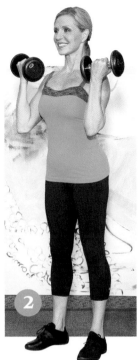

Dumbbell Curls:

Either sitting or standing, hold dumbbells in both hands with your arms at your sides. Curl one weight up until your arm is completely flexed, making sure to keep your elbows close to your sides throughout the exercise. Repeat with other arm in an alternating fashion. Conversely, you can curl both arms at the same time.

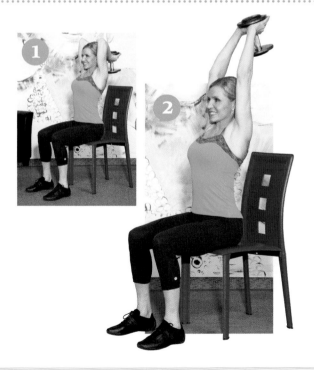

One-Dumbbell Overhead Triceps Extension:

Take hold of a dumbbell and bring back behind your head, holding one dumbbell with both hands. Extend your arms above your head until your elbows are straight. Carefully lower the weight to the start position by bending your elbows. Repeat.

Abdominal Crunches:

Lie on a mat with your hands resting under your head and your elbows out to the side. You could choose instead to cross your arms at the front of your chest. Keep your knees bent with your feet on the floor. Pick a point on the ceiling to stare at and lift your torso until your shoulder blades are off the ground. Lower to the starting position, keeping your eyes on your focus point. Be careful not to yank on your neck, and consciously use your abdominal muscles throughout the movement. Repeat.

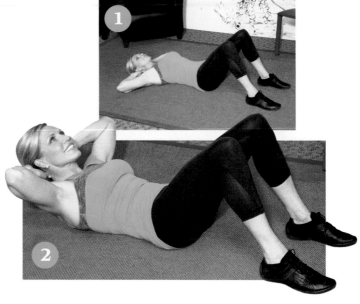

Supermans:

Lie on your stomach on the floor. Extend your arms out in front of you and keep your legs straight. Lift your legs and arms off the ground simultaneously. Hold for one to five seconds. Return to the starting position and repeat.

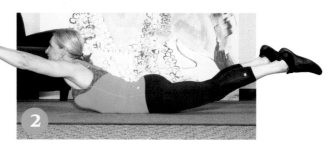

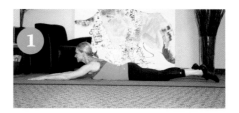

Bicycle Crunches:

Lie on a mat with your hands resting under your head and your elbows out to the side. Lifting your legs off the ground, rotate your torso, bringing your left knee and right elbow toward each other. At the same time straighten your right leg, keeping the foot off the floor. Do the same on the opposite side, and then alternate back and forth in a fluid motion. Be careful not to yank on your neck.

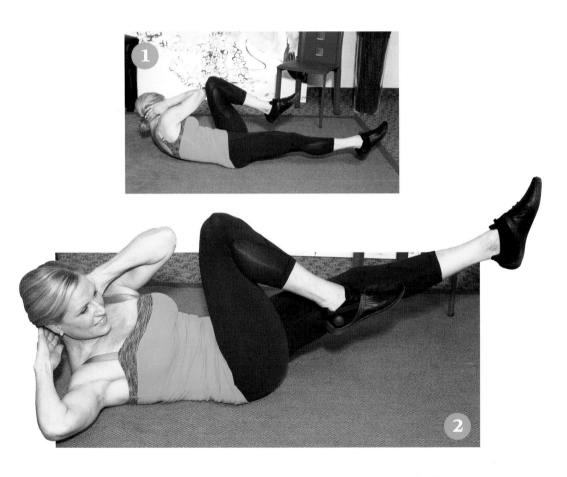

"Be careful not to yank on your neck."

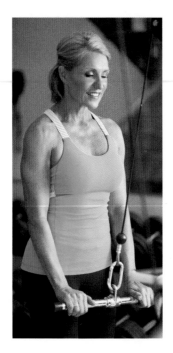

Stay *Stripped* with a Switch

Muscle memory can wreak havoc on your goals. Just when you think you are making progress, you discover your muscles have gotten the better of you and have adapted to the stress you have been throwing at them during your resistance training. You find it easier to accomplish your exercises and you're just not getting the results you want. It's time to change your routine and increase the intensity. This can be done in a number of ways, including changing the exercise you use to hit the muscle, increasing the weight or changing the number of sets and repetitions. You can find alternative exercises for each of the ones in this chapter at www.eatcleandiet.com/changeitup.

Busting Out of the Rut: Change the Weight

Increase the amount of weight you are lifting to fit your strength. If you were using 10 pounds in each hand for your biceps curls, try increasing the weight to 12 or 15 pounds. You want to feel challenged by the last repetition without losing correct training form. You will likely have to lower the number of reps you are doing when you first increase the weight. That's okay! Work your way back up in reps before increasing the weight again.

Busting Out of the Rut: Change the Repetitions and Sets

You can increase the number of repetitions and sets until you reach exhaustion. Most people start by performing eight reps per set. You can work your way up to doing as many as 20 reps per set depending on the exercise. Remember to maintain proper form.

"You find it easier to accomplish your exercises and you're just not getting the results you want. It's time to change your routine and increase the intensity."

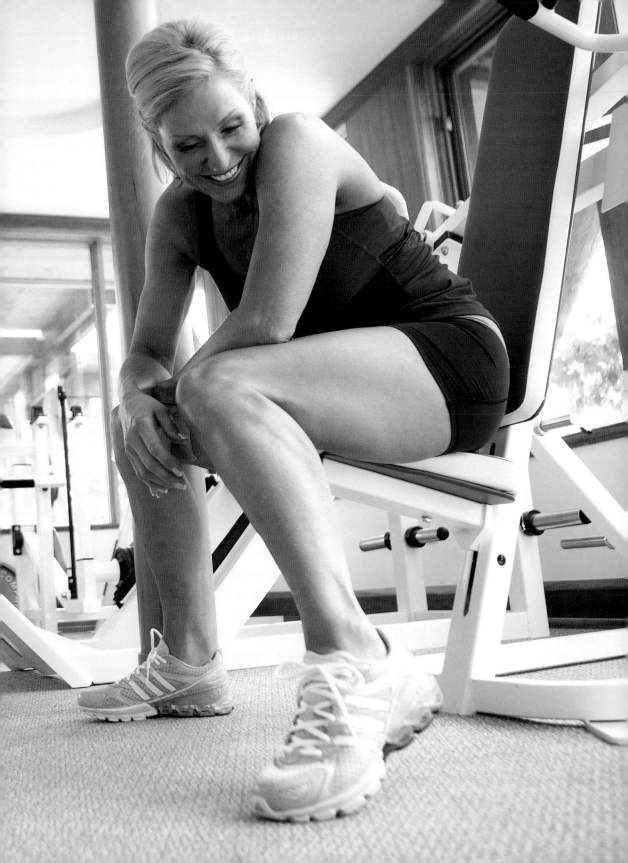

▶ Protein and Protein Supplements

IF YOU ASK ANY PHYSIQUE ENTHUSIAST what the most important nutrient is for putting on muscle you will get a unanimous response: protein! Protein is useful for you, the weight-loss enthusiast, because you are interested in building lean muscle to drive up your metabolic rate and protein is that necessary building block. The question for you is: what kind of protein supplement should you use and when?

Types of Protein Supplements

Numerous kinds of protein supplements exist, many of which are targeted to athletes, bodybuilders, hardgainers and of course, you the dieter. Generally, protein powders contain 20 to 30 grams of protein per serving and come in a variety of flavors. Most supplements contain protein from whey, casein, egg, soy, rice and hemp.

Whey:

Whey protein is one of the most popular protein supplements because it is inexpensive and excellent for muscle building and repair immediately following a workout. It is a by-product of making dairy products such as cheese. The benefit of this protein source is that it is easily digested, breaking down in about one hour. If you're lactose intolerant you are better off choosing a whey protein isolate as it assimilates rapidly into the body.

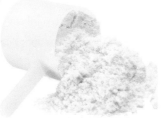

Casein:

Casein protein, also made from milk, can take up to seven hours to digest and is therefore called a slow-digesting protein. It is popular among weight gainers who drink it at night to avoid catabolism (muscle breakdown that occurs in part because of inadequate nutrition). It can be quite costly because of its high protein content (92 percent) and high contents of glutamine and amino acid favored by the brain and important to hormone balance.

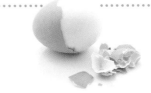

Egg:

Egg protein (albumin) is derived from egg whites and is ideal for lactose-intolerant individuals and those with milk allergies. This was a very popular protein supplement at one time but is no longer very common. It can be found in powdered form, and is also incorporated into many supplements such as protein bars and meal replacements. This protein is fairly inexpensive and takes approximately one to three hours to digest.

Soy:

Soy protein is popular among vegetarians and individuals who are lactose-intolerant and/or allergic to milk or egg products. It is considered a complete protein because soya beans contain all nine essential amino acids. It is a fast-digesting protein. Whether or not one should use soy protein is a controversial subject. Studies show that soy supplements can alleviate pre- and post-menopausal symptoms while lowering the risk of breast cancer, and that encourages use. However, because soy acts as a phytoestrogen some people question whether it might actually encourage cancer growth and whether it is good for muscle building.

Rice:

A valuable alternative protein source for vegetarians and/or lactose-intolerant individuals is rice protein. It is gluten free and low in fat, sugar and carbohydrates. This type of protein is highly unlikely to cause any allergic reactions and contains fiber, which helps lower cholesterol and curb hunger.

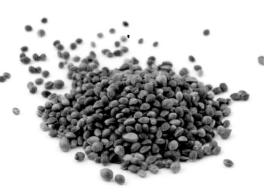

Hemp:

Another excellent source of protein is hemp protein. The protein found in hemp is similar to protein found in the human body. Not only does hemp protein provide essential fatty acids, but it is also an excellent source of dietary fiber. This plant protein also provides antioxidants, vitamins, minerals and chlorophyll. Hemp protein is vegan, gluten free, non-genetically modified (non-GMO) and is usually kosher.

Why Do You Need A Protein Supplement?

In *The Eat-Clean Diet Stripped* we are working hard to help you shed excess weight. Part of your success involves Eating Clean, which means you are to eat six small meals each day and include both a complex carbohydrate and a protein at each meal. Sometimes the quickest and most convenient way to do this is to depend on liquid meals in the form of shakes and smoothies. In either of these it is a simple matter to measure out a scoop of your favorite protein source and combine a few other ingredients in a blender. Press the button and in minutes you will have a delicious, protein-packed beverage to help you stay on track. Try out some of the following recipes to help you stick to your *Stripped* plan. Results are sure to follow.

Pre-Workout Pineapple Blast Shake

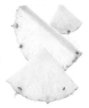

INGREDIENTS

4 ice cubes

1 cup / 240 ml water

1 scoop vanilla whey protein powder

½ cup / 120 ml pineapple chunks

METHOD

1 Process all ingredients in a blender until mixed thoroughly and serve.

Ultra Chocolate Oatmeal Shake

INGREDIENTS

½ cup / 120 ml precooked plain oatmeal

1 scoop chocolate protein powder

½ cup / 120 ml skim or almond milk

METHOD

1 Process all of the ingredients in a blender until mixed thoroughly and serve.

Yummy Banana Soy Shake

INGREDIENTS

1 banana

1 scoop soy vanilla protein powder

1 Tbsp / 15 ml almond butter

1 Tbsp / 15 ml wheat germ

½ cup / 120 ml skim or almond milk

METHOD

1 Process all ingredients in a blender until mixed thoroughly and serve.

Chocolate Strawberry Dream Shake

INGREDIENTS

1 scoop chocolate protein powder

¾ cup / 180 ml water

4 ice cubes

8 strawberries

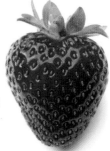

METHOD

1 Process all ingredients in a blender for one minute. Pour into a tall glass and garnish with a strawberry.

Orange Creamsicle Shake

INGREDIENTS

1 scoop vanilla protein powder

½ cup / 120 ml water

4 ice cubes

1 orange, peeled

¼ cup / 60 ml skim or almond milk

METHOD

1 Process all ingredients in a blender until well blended. Garnish with an orange wheel.

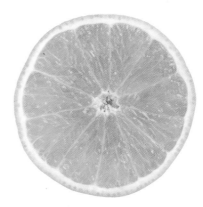

Very-Berry Blaster

INGREDIENTS

1 scoop strawberry protein powder

½ cup / 120 ml water

4 ice cubes

½ cup / 120 ml blueberries

½ cup / 120 ml raspberries

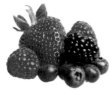

METHOD

1 Process all ingredients in a blender for one minute or until well blended.

"Pick Me Up" Energy Shake

INGREDIENTS

¾ cup / 180 ml water

10 strawberries

1 Tbsp / 15 ml flaxseed oil

1 scoop chocolate, vanilla or strawberry protein powder

¼ tsp / 1.25 ml agave nectar

1 tsp / 5 ml wheat germ

METHOD

1 Process all ingredients in a blender to desired consistency. Garnish with a strawberry.

Oatmeal Meal Replacement Shake

INGREDIENTS

½ cup / 120 ml cooked oatmeal

1 scoop vanilla protein powder

⅛ tsp / pinch cinnamon

¼ tsp / 1.25 ml agave nectar

1 Tbsp / 15 ml chopped almonds or natural nut butter

¾ cup / 180 ml almond milk or water

METHOD

1 Place all ingredients in a blender and blend to desired consistency. Drink your meal!

Light and Healthy Hemp Protein Shake

INGREDIENTS

1 scoop organic hemp protein

1 cup / 240 ml water

1 banana

½ cup / 120 ml blueberries

1 tsp / 5 ml wheat germ

METHOD

1 Process all ingredients in a blender to desired consistency. Pour into a tall glass and enjoy!

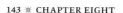

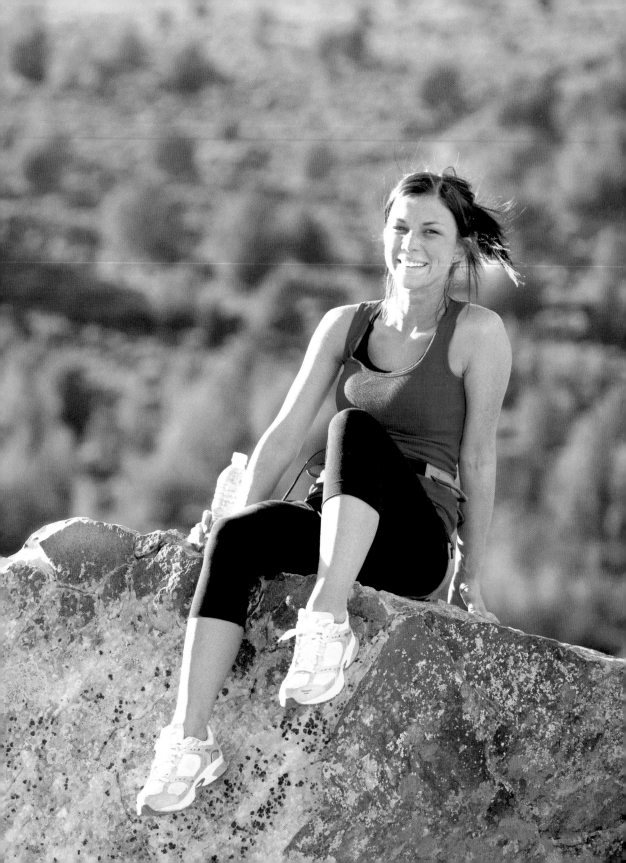

9 | Take the Next Step

he first step of any journey is often the most difficult, but it also can be the easiest. Yes, making the decision to change your nutritional ways is a big step, but once you've made it and start your new relationship with food, you enter a "honeymoon period" similar to when you begin a new loving relationship. You wake up happy and energized, looking forward to feeding your body a new sort of food – Clean food. Everything feels right and the future is rosy. And for some, as with some marriages, this feeling seems to last forever.

> **"To achieve your goals and remain successful, you must be willing to step over the line and fully commit to change."**

Many people, however, will at some point notice their commitment waning. You may find your perspective changing; instead of looking at what you are getting from your new relationship with food, such as a lean body, an improved sex life, balanced mood and hormones, beautiful skin and hair, clear eyes and tons of energy, you begin focusing on what you can't have – nachos and margaritas with the gang, drive-thru burgers, fries and soda.

This is where the yo-yo experience of losing and gaining weight often begins. You lose 10 or 20 pounds, slip back to your old habits and then find yourself back where you started – or possibly even heavier. This is also where you're likely to stop within reach of your goal, never quite having reached it. You see the finish line and choke instead of running for it. This is called self-sabotage.

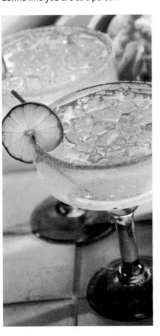

▼ **YOUR OLD HABITS,** such as going out for drinks and junk food, don't define who you are as a person.

To achieve your goals and remain successful, you must be willing to step over the line and fully commit to change, and that can be scary. You have an idea of yourself and the way you live your life that is comfortable to you. Like a ratty old pair of slippers or an unattractive pair of jeans, you put this comfortable persona on each day out of habit. This habit ends up being how you define yourself and how others see you. You are the person who drinks margaritas and eats nachos with the gang. You are the person who hates shopping for new clothes because you would rather not see the bulges. You are the person who takes your kids to a drive thru on the way to soccer practice. Now is the time to realize these are not definitions of who you are; they are simply habits you've had up until this point. These are the habits you will now change. You won't break free and grab that brass ring of success until you stop defining yourself in this way.

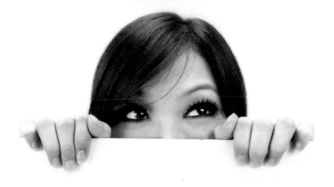

AVOIDING SELF-SABOTAGE
Fear of Success

Here is a scenario that may be familiar to you. A woman wants
to lose 15 pounds. She starts a diet and sticks to it faithfully. After
two weeks she feels lighter and her pants are getting loose. She
finds she's lost five pounds. Yes! This makes her feel great. She
goes shopping and, hardly thinking about it, picks up a candy
bar. She doesn't really know why she's picking it up, but tells
herself it's a treat. That night at dinner she adds butter to her
potatoes and gets a second helping of food. The next morning she
eats an omelet loaded with cheese and fats, served alongside a big
plate of home fries. She can spare a few extra calories, right? She
lost five pounds! But by the end of the weekend she's regained all
of her lost weight. Sure, much of this is water, but she doesn't
really think about that. The number on the scale says the same
number it did two weeks ago. Discouraged that all the hard work
can be erased so quickly, she gives up and settles back into her old
ways. This is a scenario that is played out all over North America
millions of times a day.

This woman displays classic "fear of success" behavior. As soon as
she began to reach her goals, she – without conscious thought –
made sure she didn't reach them. If this sounds familiar to you,
then you might need to dig deep and excavate the reason you fear
success. Maybe you are comfortable fading into the woodwork,
and you fear the attention you might get if you create a killer

> "You might
> need to dig
> deep and
> excavate the
> reason you
> fear success."

> "Maybe you fear the attention you might get if you create a killer body."

body. Maybe your mother makes unkind comments about some people being "too skinny" and you don't want people making comments like that about you. But the most common reason people experience fear of success is, ironically, their fear of failure.

The fear of success credo might go something like this: "If I really try to achieve a goal and don't do it, then I will have failed. If I don't really try to succeed, then I won't have failed." Sounds kind of silly when you put it that way, doesn't it? In reality, this prevents many people from succeeding because they see trying hard at something as being risky.

You have to risk possible failure by trying, perhaps that's true, but you are *guaranteed* failure by *not* trying! As the Great One, Wayne Gretzky, once said, "You miss 100 percent of the shots you don't take." Besides, those who are truly successful understand that failure is an integral part of success. The persistent inventor Thomas Alva Edison famously said about his idea for a light bulb: "I have not failed. I've just found 10,000 ways that won't work." He never considered giving up and now we have him to thank when we switch on a light by which to read.

No one does everything perfectly all the time, although it may sometimes appear that others do when you're watching them from the outside. Success does not come from perfection; it comes from consistently moving in the right direction, which eventually brings you where you want to be, and that is something you really don't need to fear.

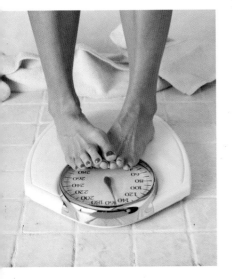

▼ **DON'T LET YOUR** fear of failure stand in the way of your goals. You are your biggest obstacle!

Fear of Change

Achieving a weight-loss goal, by definition, means you will change both your eating behavior and the way you look and feel. Noticeable alterations in these departments will also transform your body, perhaps dramatically. While these adjustments may be desirable to you, (think about the goals you set for yourself in your journal), the change itself can be frightening and difficult. We develop behavioral habits and patterns that quickly become the comfort zone out of which we operate all the time. Like that old ratty pair of slippers and baggy jeans, we wear our habits and follow our behavioral patterns even though we deserve better. And you do deserve better! The trick is to step out of your comfort zone into a brand new arena.

Habits can be difficult to break, but they are easy to form. That means you can replace old negative habits with positive new ones without too much difficulty. Yes, it will take a bit of effort on your part, but according to many experts on behavior modification, it takes only 28 days for a new habit to form and stick. That's less than one month to get rid of your bad habits for good!

If you normally eat dinner and then flake out on the couch eating cookies and watching TV, then start going for a walk every night after dinner. In a few short weeks you will have replaced a negative habit with a positive one. Don't leave yourself empty; make sure to always give yourself a positive replacement habit for every negative habit you are changing. You may be able to make these changes all at once or it might work better for you to change one bad habit at a time. I'm an all-or-nothing kind of girl, and that means when I make a decision to do something I dive in headfirst. Slow, gradual changes don't work for me. Each of us is different in this respect, and for some people diving in would

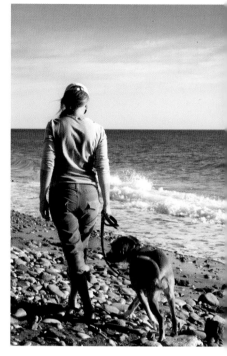

▲ **THINK OF YOUR** daily walk as a luxury – time where you can reflect on the positive changes you're making.

"The most common reason people experience fear of success is, ironically, their fear of failure."

> "Another great way to deal with these physical changes is to envision them before they occur."

never work. Don't guess at where on this spectrum you lie. Look at your past successes and how you accomplished them, and make your decision from there. Jump in if you are fearless. Take your time if that is the better way for you. Neither is wrong and both will give you that 10-pounds-lighter body.

If you have a hard time dealing with the physical changes in your body, try not to focus on them. When you are following the Eat-Clean Diet lifestyle you have a lot more to think about than just your shrinking waistline. You are creating a whole new healthy life for yourself! Start learning about the healthiest foods and what they offer you. Search for local farmers' markets. Challenge yourself to make meals using the freshest in-season ingredients, or try one new food each week. Make each meal as nutritious as possible. If you follow the Eat-Clean Diet Principles and specifically the plan within this book, then you don't have to worry about whether or not you're losing weight – the weight will come off.

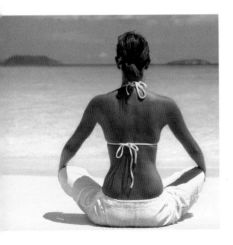

Another great way to deal with these physical changes is to envision them before they occur. Every morning and evening, close your eyes and picture yourself with the body you're trying to achieve. Picture yourself looking down and seeing a flat tummy, a small waistline. Visualize yourself walking on a beach wearing a bikini, without a jiggle to be seen. Visualization is a powerful success technique that hearkens back to what we discussed earlier – your idea of yourself. If the way you want to be is not in sync with the way you see yourself, then you'd better change the way you see yourself!

Sabotage By Others

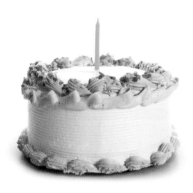

It's bad enough that we have to deal with our own issues surrounding success and change, but the sad truth is that we have to deal with the fears of those around us as well. From a co-worker who brings a box of donuts into the office every meeting to the loving aunt who invites you over for a deep-fried dinner to a husband who wants to continue vegging out in front of the TV with you and a shared pint of Haagen-Dazs each evening ... saboteurs are everywhere. Even your own children can stand against you while you strive to make change. It can be daunting and off-putting but you want results, so here is how to handle the nay sayers.

Sometimes these people are well-meaning, such as Ashley in the web department who lives on junk food because her metabolism is still on youthful fire – she thinks she's being a nice co-worker when she brings in a box of Krispy Kremes. The most hurtful sabotage I experienced in my physique transformation came from my children. We were celebrating a birthday along with the predictable birthday cake heavy with icing. As we sang the birthday song, my children taunted me, questioning whether or not I would eat the cake. One of them smeared the icing on my nose. I felt hurt by that but I understood they were expressing a fear that Mom was going to be different and they didn't like it. I ate a bit of icing and cake but stuck to my own plan of wanting to be a slimmer, healthier me.

You may encounter none of these types of sabotage, or you may encounter all and more. Be warned: some sort of sabotage will come your way, so be prepared ahead of time on how you'll deal with it or that sabotage will work – meaning you won't reach your goals.

> "Be warned: some sort of sabotage will come your way, so be prepared ahead of time on how you'll deal with it."

> "The mental fortitude that comes along with real commitment is strong."

To avoid being sidelined, the first step you'll have to take is to be fully committed to your dietary changes and weight loss. Being committed makes it easier, because the mental fortitude that comes along with real commitment is strong. If you go to your meeting with Ashley saying to yourself, "I am committed to my new diet and lifestyle. It doesn't matter if there are donuts there. I've made a commitment and I'm sticking to it," the results will be quite different than if you say, "I want to lose those last 10 pounds but Ashley always brings donuts in and they always taste so good. I'll try to resist them."

You have to prepare yourself ahead of time, both mentally and physically. You can mentally prepare by reminding yourself of your commitment. Your physical preparation comes from eating something Clean before your meeting. If you are starving you'll have a much harder time resisting donuts than if you have a belly full of Clean food.

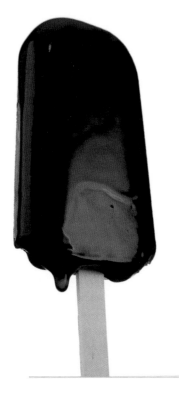

▼ **INSTEAD OF ICE CREAM AND CANDY** try dessert-flavored herbal teas to satisfy your sweet tooth.

Just because your husband loves the time spent with you eating ice cream does not mean he won't love doing something else with you instead. You could replace ice cream with tea. You could ask him to join you for an after-dinner walk, join a ballroom dance class, a bowling league or a gym. The solution is not to simply take away the bad habit; it's to replace the bad habit with a good one. If he balks, have a heart-to-heart with him. Tell him how important it is to you that you succeed, and ask him for his help.

How you act with your deep-fried food-loving aunt will depend very much on her reasons for giving you this food and on your relationship with her. Some possible solutions might be to let her know ahead of time that you are on a strict eating plan and that you love to spend time with her, but will bring your own food to eat. This reasoning often goes over better if you make it a health issue rather than a weight issue. You could tell her, for example, that you have discovered some food intolerances and have to be very careful what you eat. Who can argue with that?

These are just some suggestions and obviously you will have to develop your own solutions to deal with the saboteurs that come your way. The point is that you do have to have a solution to this potential problem if you want to succeed. When you go in with commitment and a game plan, you *will* succeed – there's no question.

Maintenance – Yo-Yo No More!

In order to take the next step and lose those last 10 pounds you need to make the commitment, have a plan and allow yourself to succeed. The same is true once you have achieved that goal and wish to stay there. Maintaining your weight loss can be difficult if you don't have a strategy. All too often we lose the weight, reach our goal and say, "Great, now I can get back to eating normally!" Of course, getting back to eating "normally" means going back to your old "normal" weight. Such a mindset will not keep you lean for long. Staying at a reduced bodyweight doesn't happen all on its own. At the same time, you cannot stay on your same weight-loss plan; you don't want to keep losing weight. This is when you should progress to the "Cooler 2" plan. I will give you the basics for this plan here, but it is outlined in more depth in *The Eat-Clean Diet Recharged!* You will want to ease your way into following Cooler 2 so you don't gain any weight back. Increase your starchy carbs, for example, a little at a time. But make your mind up now! After you finish the *Stripped* program you will not gain those 10 pounds right back. You'll keep them off forever with your changed new outlook, and the Cooler 2 plan.

▼ "COOLER 2" is my lifestyle way of eating. It is both for weight loss and weight maintenance.

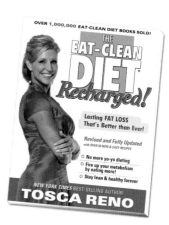

What it's for:

1 Steady weight loss.

2 Maintenance once your goal weight is reached. Cooler 2 may not be enough for the stubborn last 10. If you have more than 10 to lose or if you are ready to maintain your weight loss, this plan is for you.

Why it works:

When your body begins approaching its set point (its genetically predetermined healthy weight), you will find that weight loss will slow or stop. That's why you need the *Stripped* plan to lose those last few pounds, and that is why the Cooler 2 plan works for maintenance, even though it works for weight loss when you are heavier.

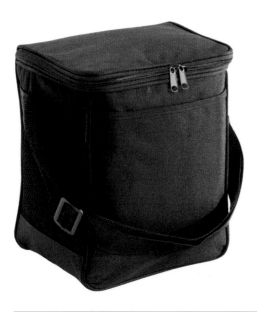

COOLER 2 IN DETAIL

Lean Protein:

5 – 6 portions each day. A portion is:

✳ 1 cup/handful of low-fat or nonfat dairy products (soy, almond, hemp, rice or lactose-free milk, cottage cheese, kefir, plain yogurt, Yogurt Cheese*)

✳ 1 scant handful of raw, unsalted nuts

✳ 2 tablespoons of natural nut butter

✳ 1 palm-sized portion of lean meat

✳ Natural (sugar- and chemical-free) protein powder (hemp, soy or whey)

✳ Vegetarian protein sources (see page 94)

*Yogurt Cheese recipe, see page 301.

Complex Carbohydrates from Fruit and Vegetables:

6 portions each day. A portion is:

✳ 1 cupped handful or piece of fruit, especially berries, grapefruit, melons, bananas, apples, mangoes

✳ 2 cupped handfuls of vegetables including broth-based/vegetable purée soups

Complex Carbohydrates from Whole Grains and Starchy Carbohydrates:

2 to 4 portions each day. A portion is:

✳ 1 scant handful of high-protein, sugar-free cold cereals, such as muesli and granola

✳ 1 handful of cooked cereal

✳ 1 piece of whole grain bread or seven-inch wrap

✳ 1 handful-sized serving of sweet potato, yam, corn, carrots and squash

Beverages:

2 to 3 liters per day of fresh water with no sodium.

✳ Caffeine-free herbal tea

✳ Black coffee (in moderation)

✳ Green/black tea

Sweeteners:

Use these in moderation.

Avoid artificial sweeteners.

✳ Honey

✳ Agave nectar

✳ Stevia

✳ Sucanat

✳ Rapadura sugar

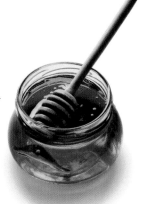

Healthy Fats:

2 to 3 servings each day. A serving is:

✳ 1 to 2 Tbsp of oils, especially olive, pumpkin-seed, flaxseed and safflower

✳ 1 to 2 Tbsp nut butters

✳ 1 scant handful unsalted, raw nuts

✳ 1 to 2 Tbsp olive-oil based spreads

✳ Fish and fish oils

Avoid:

✘ Juice

✘ Commercial salad dressings or sauces

✘ Fried, refined and processed foods

In order to maintain your weight loss with this Cooler 2 plan, you will eat carefully and choose your foods well, but you will not eat as strictly as you did in order to blast through the 10 pounds you are working on now.

As I stated earlier, you do not want to jump right into Cooler 2. Your body has been through a super-strict period while losing those last 10 pounds, and jumping to the carbohydrates and fats in Cooler 2 would likely be counterproductive. Ease your way into it over a couple of weeks. Give your body a chance to adjust. Add one serving of carbohydrates every day or two, rotating fruit, starches and formerly forbidden vegetables, until you reach the actual Cooler 2 limits. Do the same for fats and also dairy products if you eat them.

Treats During Maintenance

If you are trying to keep your new body (and why wouldn't you?) then treats are fine, as long as they are just that – treats. If you have a small ice cream, a glass of wine or a little bit of dark chocolate once a week as a treat while following the Cooler 2 plan the rest of the time along with doing regular exercise, you should have no problem staying within a couple of pounds of your ideal weight. If you start having one of these treats every day, then they are no longer treats but instead part of your everyday diet. It's always your choice what you eat, how much and how often. But keep in mind that if you have treats too often you may not like the results.

Remember that *The Eat-Clean Diet* is not really a "diet" in the traditional sense of that word. It is a lifestyle way of eating that helps you eat more nutritiously, but helps you lose weight producing a healthy, fit body. It quickly becomes your way of life and before long you will be appalled at the food you used to eat.

◀ **WHEN TEMPTED** by treats, visualize yourself reaching your goals, and then decide if having that treat is worth it.

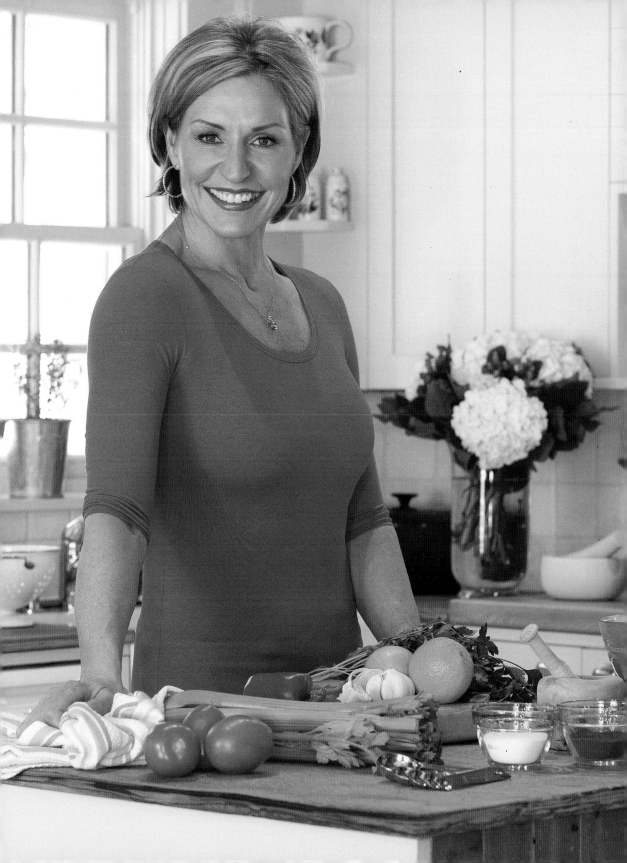

Drink to Get *Stripped*!

Staying hydrated is critical to strip off the last few pounds. Your body is 60 to 70 percent water. This amount is determined by the amount of fat and muscle you carry. Muscle is made of approximately 90 percent water, while fat is only 20 percent water. This means the more muscle you have, the more water you'll carry.

When you are dehydrated your muscles lose elasticity – this can happen within a 30-minute workout session. When muscles lose elasticity they lose their ability to work properly, causing cramps and spasms and decreasing their ability to burn calories. Muscle definition also depends on water, so if you are looking for tone it is essential to stay hydrated.

Water is necessary for all bodily functions. You can live without food but you can't last long without water. Digestion is dependant on water. Dehydration can cause constipation and damage to your GI tract and stomach lining.

Dehydration is also responsible for daytime fatigue, headaches and joint pain. When you are deprived of water, your body shuts down. So drink up – you will become more energized in your everyday activities and have better workout results. It's as easy as reaching for a glass of water at every meal.

The following *Stripped* drink options will help you stay hydrated on your weight-loss mission. Blends of spices, herbs, fruits and vegetables have been created to optimize weight loss – and taste delicious.

Metabolism: The herbs and spices in this smoothie stimulate your metabolism.

Burn, Baby Burn Smoothie

INGREDIENTS

1 cup / 240 ml tomato juice
¼ tsp / 1.25 ml black pepper
Pinch cayenne pepper
Pinch cinnamon
Pinch cumin
¼ tsp / 1.25 ml ground ginger
¼ tsp / 1.25 ml turmeric

METHOD

1 Blend all ingredients and serve.

TIP: Quench your thirst and your cravings. We often confuse thirst and hunger, so try drinking a glass of water before reaching for that chocolate bar. On second thought, don't reach for a chocolate bar – try one of the delicious recipes in this book!

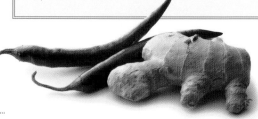

Digestion: The ingredients and combinations in this recipe help relieve gas and nausea, and ease the digestion of carbohydrates and fiber.

Digestion Doozey Smoothie

INGREDIENTS

1 cup / 240 ml coconut water
¼ tsp / 1.25 ml black pepper
¼ tsp / 1.25 ml celery seed
¼ tsp / 1.25 ml fennel seeds
1 clove garlic
Handful fresh mint
2 Tbsp / 30 ml fresh oregano
1 Tbsp / 15 ml fresh sage
½ tsp / 2.5 ml fresh thyme

METHOD

1 Blend all ingredients and serve.

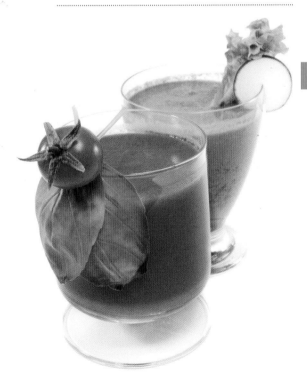

Appetite, Weight Loss and Cravings: This blend is targeted to reduce appetite through hydration and spices.

Helping Hunger Smoothie

INGREDIENTS:

1 cup / 240 ml coconut water
10 fresh basil leaves
Pinch cayenne pepper
¼ tsp / 1.25 ml cinnamon
1 clove garlic
Pinch ground ginger

METHOD

1 Blend all ingredients and serve.

Colds, Headaches and Stomach Aches: This drink will cover

everything from stomach aches, bloat, vomiting and nausea to a runny nose.

Immune Protection in a Cup

INGREDIENTS

1 cup / 240 ml water or coconut water
Pinch cardamom
Pinch cayenne pepper
¼ tsp / 1.25 ml fennel seeds
1 clove garlic
Pinch ground ginger
¼ tsp / 1.25 ml mustard seed
Handful fresh mint leaves
1 Tbsp / 15 ml fresh oregano
1 Tbsp / 15 ml raw honey

METHOD

1 Blend all ingredients and serve.

> **For more *Stripped* drinks, visit:**
> www.eatcleandiet.com/yourstrippeddrinks

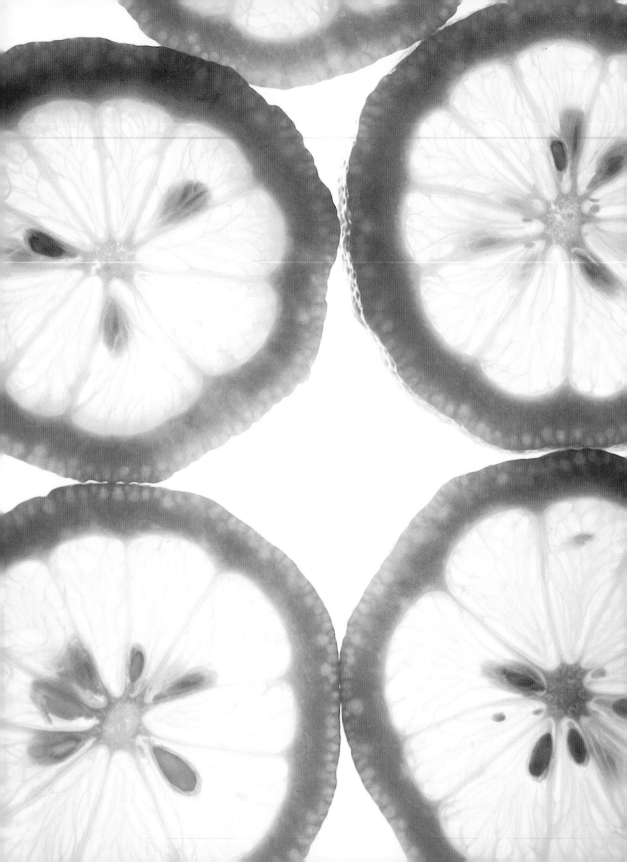

10 | Tricks of the Trade

The Eat-Clean Diet is by definition a detoxification diet since the word itself means cleansing toxins from the body as well as from your mind. The Eat Clean Diet urges choosing minimally processed foods and avoiding all chemically charged, toxin-laden foods. Our society culturally accepts the need to cleanse the body periodically, but there is no reason to torture yourself with a limited diet of lemon water mixed with maple syrup and spices. Simply starting to Eat Clean by following the Principles of this practical lifestyle way of eating will cause your body to undergo a cleanse. This alone may be all you need to shed that final 10 pounds. Exciting, isn't it?

Putting Detox Into Perspective

Your body is perfectly equipped to accomplish cleansing and detoxification – think liver, heart, lungs, kidneys, skin, digestive tract and lymph nodes. Today, however, these organs are under assault from pollution and chemicals and have become inundated with toxins. The modern lifestyle has accelerated into overdrive, so you may also be dealing with heightened stress levels. If you participate in risky behaviors, including alcohol abuse and the use of recreational drugs, your body will be begging for a cleanse.

"If you participate in risky behaviors ... your body will be begging for a cleanse."

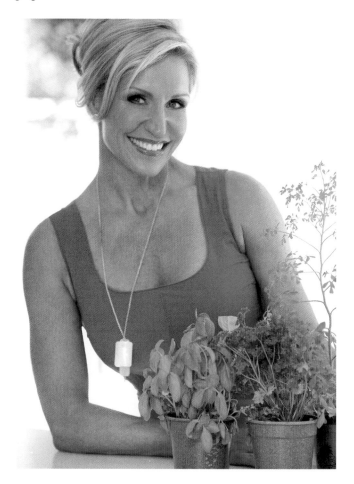

Eat Clean and Detox

Combining the power of *The Eat-Clean Diet* with a few more cleansing habits will step up your rate of weight loss. I've adopted the habit of starting each day with a cleansing beverage. As soon as I wake up and have wiggled my feet into my slippers, I head for the kitchen, where I reach for a lemon. I roll the fruit on the counter to help it release some of its valuable juice (my Dad taught me this trick), slice the lemon in half and squeeze out as much fresh juice as possible into a large glass. To this I add hot water and sip this refreshing beverage before I do anything else. This drink is said to assist with cleansing the liver as well as the bowels. As toxins disappear from the body the skin also perfects itself. Drinking lemon water will help you get rid of blemishes.

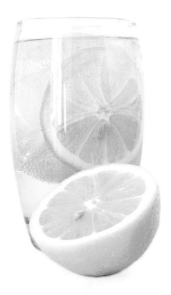

Some of you may have heard of the "Master Cleanse." It is similar to the mixture I recommend – lemon juice and water – but adds one tablespoon of maple syrup and a pinch of cayenne pepper and/or ginger. Since you are interested in shedding those last 10 pounds I recommend drinking plain water with a shot of lemon juice and no additives. The maple syrup would be counter-productive to your goal of wanting to lose weight. Though natural, maple syrup is still a sugar and can be stored as fat.

Set the Tone

After drinking your lemon water you have set the tone for the day. I always feel better after I have had this drink and it helps me stick with my Eat-Clean plans all day; I don't want to spoil things by eating junk. Let this hot lemon-water drink be your starting point too. Practice it every day.

BENEFITS OF DRINKING LEMON WATER EACH DAY

→ Helps shed toxins from the body

→ Acts as a liver tonic

→ Improves skin tone and quality

→ Works as a natural diuretic

→ Helps dissolve gallstones

→ Breaks down phlegm

→ Relieves nausea

→ Relieves constipation

→ Is a digestive aid

→ Alkalizes the body

→ Improves immunity

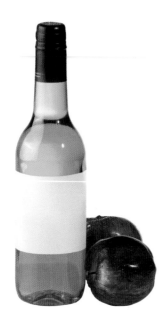

APPLE CIDER VINEGAR:

Organic apple cider vinegar, called ACV, is also useful when trying to lose weight, because the vinegar helps shorten the time fats linger in your digestive tract. The less time fats spend being digested, the less chance they will be stored as fat. ACV also helps the body burn fat and fuel more efficiently by releasing iron from what we eat, which in turn causes more oxygen to be used, helping you lose weight. Like lemon juice, apple cider vinegar has a cleansing quality, particularly because organic ACV, which includes "the mother" (unfiltered product – the part with the most health benefits), has potent antibiotic and antiseptic characteristics. Try drinking two tablespoons of ACV mixed into a glass of water daily.

▲ **PURCHASE** apple cider vinegar at some grocery stores and most health-food stores.

Physical Activity for Detox

Physical activity enhances the elimination of waste and toxins. I remember taking my young daughters to the zoo one day to have "Breakfast with the Elephants," a hugely popular event. Mothers and small children crowded around to see the big animals. Before the elephants could eat they were to have a bath, but first they had to "walk the perimeter." The trainers had found through experience that when the elephants walked several laps around the pool it would get the pachyderms' digestive tracts moving. This way large deposits (and there were many) didn't end up in the pool. Soon afterwards the elephants were let loose in the water and the fun began. The point is that exercise makes your digestive tract move over and above its normal activity. Exercise facilitates your detoxification process just as it does for the elephants. Of course an increased intake of water and fiber – according to the Eat-Clean Diet Principles – also encourages the cleansing process.

"Exercise makes your digestive tract move over and above its normal activity."

More About Elimination: Flaxseed

People who know me well know I'm an emphatic cheerleader when it comes to flaxseed. Before experiencing the power of Eating Clean, I was a terrible eliminator. My bowels were lazy, and in that respect I was keeping company with two-thirds of the North American population. It is important to realize how dangerous constipation can be for your health. When fecal matter remains in the bowel for too long, the delicate tissues of the colon come in contact with potentially lethal toxins. Worse still, the fecal matter can build up in the colon, becoming cement-like. Over time it becomes more and more difficult to eliminate and the colon can become impacted, requiring surgery to relieve the situation.

Why not avoid all this trouble by adding something simple, natural and inexpensive to your diet? Just eat two tablespoons of ground flaxseed every day. I buy the seeds whole and grind them at home in a coffee grinder, then store the ground seeds in a glass jar in the refrigerator. The seeds must be ground to a coarse meal in order to be digested properly. Flaxseed contains loads of fiber, both soluble and insoluble, which helps give bulk to the stool, and the healthy oils also help. Once I started Eating Clean and eating flaxseed every day, I became a regular girl! Nothing feels better. You may be carrying around a few extra pounds simply because your elimination is not regular enough. Simply eating this mighty little seed could mean a flat belly. Two tablespoons at less than 25 cents a day – I'm in!

"Simply eating this mighty little seed could mean a flat belly."

Weekend Wonder *Stripped* Leek Soup

NATURE HAS PROVIDED US with certain foods that have their own weight-loss power; one of these foods is leeks. Related to garlic and onions, leeks are valued for their healthful qualities, particularly their ability to cleanse the body. They are also known for their diuretic power and that is where they come into play for you, the Eat-Clean dieter, planning to strip away those most stubborn final 10 pounds. A healthful soup made from leeks can help restore balance while encouraging the shedding of excess water (often experienced as bloat).

When I was growing up my parents always made leek soup, not only because my dad grew them in his garden, but also because they knew how nutritious these mild-onion-tasting plants were. My mother depended on leek soup to help her shed weight after her babies were born, a trick she learned from her own mother who had 13 children! My mother would drink this soup as often as she liked for a few days to help her get her body and her weight back to where it was before she became pregnant.

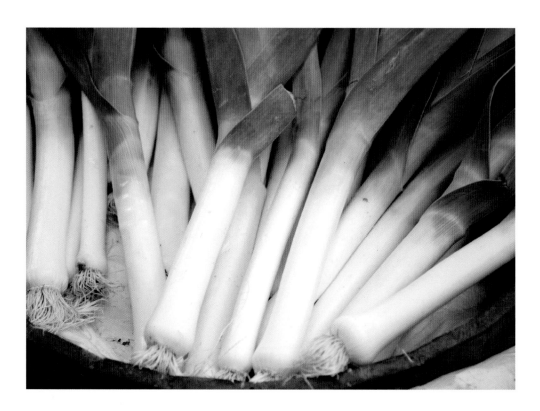

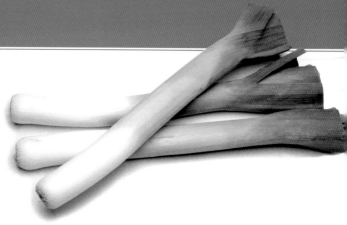

> "A healthful soup made from leeks can help restore balance while encouraging the shedding of excess water."

Apparently the Dutch and the French enjoy the same habits, as Mireille Guiliano credits a similar version of leek soup as her secret weapon for weight loss in her book, *French Women Don't Get Fat.*

French or Dutch leeks taste delicious and are inexpensive, nutritious and easy to cook. There is only one caveat: be sure to wash chopped leeks thoroughly – dirt is often trapped between the tightly packed layers.

HOW TO CHOP AND CLEAN LEEKS:

When you purchase leeks they will have an end where the roots are still attached. The other end is dark green. Begin by trimming off the root end. Then remove the darkest green part of the leek. Usually you will need to trim away about six inches of this tough green leafy part. Chop the remaining leek into rounds and place in a colander. Rinse the chopped leeks very well - use your hands to mix them so you are sure to remove all the dirt.

WEEKEND WONDER STRIPPED LEEK SOUP

1 cup / 240 ml per serving

Eat this leek soup to launch yourself into the *Stripped* plan. You will enjoy the early results – a possible weight loss of a few pounds with very little effort.

INGREDIENTS:

- **6 good-sized leeks**
- **1 fist-sized onion, peeled and coarsely chopped**
- **6 cloves garlic, peeled and passed through a garlic press**
- **6 cups / 1440 ml water**

METHOD:

1. Chop and rinse leeks (see directions below). Place rinsed leeks in a soup kettle.

2. Add chopped onion and garlic to leeks. Add 6 cups / 1440 ml water. If vegetables are not covered, add more water.

3. Bring soup to a boil on the stove. Once mixture is boiling reduce heat and let simmer for 30 minutes. Remove from heat and purée mixture using an immersion blender. Do not add seasonings or salt.

4. Serve soup hot. Store in refrigerator for three days.

Alcohol

I'm commonly asked if alcohol is part of the Eat-Clean Diet lifestyle. Alcohol intake is commonplace and has been since the birth of civilization. Unfortunately, it is often used as a tool of overindulgence. As far as I'm concerned, alcohol is just another word for sugar. An alcoholic drink is nothing but empty calories, and since we're talking detox, worst of all are its effects on your liver.

If you are trying to lose that last 10 pounds, you should avoid alcohol completely. I hear you moan, and I've heard all the excuses. Red wine is good for you ... It helps me relax ... I can't enjoy myself at a party if everyone else is drinking and I'm not ...

> "As far as I'm concerned, alcohol is just another word for sugar."

Now is the time to think about your goals. Ask yourself what is more important: having that glass of wine or meeting your goals and looking/feeling your best? I'm not saying that you must give up alcohol forever, but if you are struggling to lose that last bit of weight, you need to reevaluate your priorities.

When I'm trying to lose a few pounds I don't touch alcohol, and don't think that means I don't enjoy the occasional delicious glass of red wine. Notice I used the singular "glass" instead of "glasses." If you must have an alcoholic drink enjoy a glass of wine, water down your beverage by mixing it with carbonated water to create a spritzer, and drink lots of water before and after to maintain your hydration.

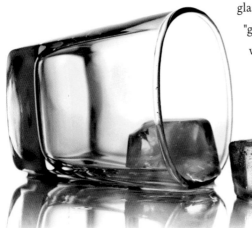

Avoiding Sodium

Too much sodium is extremely detrimental to heart health. Serious fitness pros know how important it is to keep an eye on foods that contain too much sodium before a contest – any one of these pros would be able to rhyme off a list of foods to avoid during this critical tightening-up time. Avoid all processed foods, no question. "Snacks" like chips, fries and salted nuts will derail all of the hard work you have done. To kick up your weight-loss efforts, avoid all the following foods: preserved meats including bacon and deli meats, hot dogs, pepperoni, sardines, cheese, commercial peanut butter, TV dinners, most canned foods,

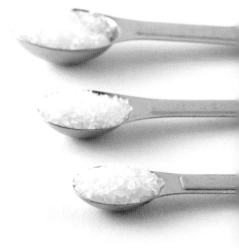

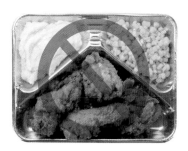

pickled vegetables, olives, relish, sauces and spreads, seasonings, vegetable juices, pasta sauce, breads, salty snack foods, pork, canned soups, bouillon cubes, Chinese take-out and other Chinese condiments. Most of these items would not be included in an Eat-Clean Diet lifestyle anyway, but in general you want to keep your food as Clean, and chemical- and additive-free as possible.

▲ **TOO MUCH SALT** leaves you looking and feeling bloated. Check the sodium content on all packaged foods.

Certain foods will help you stay well flushed out. Asparagus, green beans and broccoli will become very familiar vegetables as you work to shed your final pounds. Don't become exasperated by the steady diet of basic but nutritious foods. Keep imagining how amazing you are going to feel when you look at yourself in the mirror and see the brand new, stripped-of-fat version. It will be worth every mouthful!

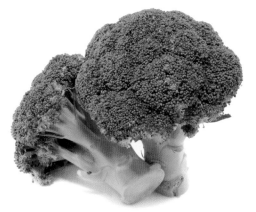

DISTILLED WATER
When Water Isn't Water

> "The tightest bodies depend on distilled water, which contains little or no sodium and reduces bloat."

Water today is not the clear liquid it once was. Food manufacturers have created numerous new concoctions of "water" containing electrolytes, protein and complex carbohydrates, to flavored waters and more. Although these sound like excellent solutions to the question of "what to drink" it pays to read labels and learn what is packed into the beverage you are about to consume. If your purpose is to lose weight you will have to be on the lookout primarily for sugar and salt. If your water tastes sweet and wonderfully delicious it is very likely filled with sugar or a sugar imposter.

Drink Distilled Water To Tighten Up in the Final Days

Regular (unflavored) water has its benefits and you can read all about them on page 60, but the tightest bodies depend on distilled water, which contains little or no sodium and reduces bloat. In your quest to shed those sticky final 10 pounds, you will want to adopt the practice of drinking distilled water to help you gain extra ground in your effort to slim down. Simply purchase or make your own distilled water and drink it from here on in. This includes your cooking water too.

Distilled Water – The Facts

Natural water contains microscopic particles along with minerals including calcium and iron. Heating this water until it becomes steam and collecting the condensed liquid is the distil-

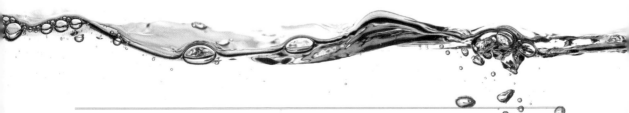

lation process that results in purified water. The resulting liquid contains only hydrogen and oxygen molecules, and has a pH of 7. All other impurities including calcium and other minerals, iron and sodium are removed during the distillation or purification process. Distilled water is pure tasting. Be aware of how your distilled water is made, and store it in inert metal containers that contribute no deleterious molecules to your body and your health; using cheap plastic containers will ruin its taste.

▼ I DRINK WATER at every one of my meals, even if I am drinking another beverage alongside it.

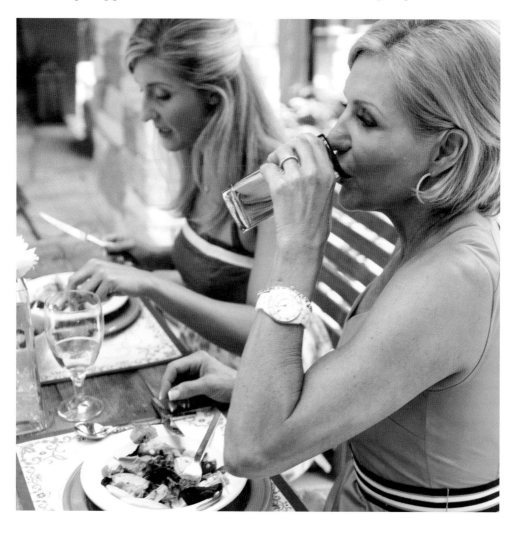

Dealing with the Detox: What is the "Cut the Crap" Hangover?

WRAPPED IN PRETTY PACKAGING and littered with scientific-sounding ingredients, junk makes up a large portion of the food North Americans eat. As soon as you "cut the crap" from your diet and start eating foods as close to nature as possible, you are on your way to a true *Eat-Clean Diet* lifestyle. A word of caution – the first few days can feel like the morning after you've had a few too many glasses of vino. A headache (among other symptoms) can crop up, leaving you in a funk, and this may deter you from maintaining your plan of renewed health. Don't give up! I can help you through this. Before you throw in the towel I want you to know that this funk is completely normal. It's called the "Cut the Crap" Hangover!

What is a "Detox?"

When you start *The Eat-Clean Diet* you induce a total body detoxification, whereby built-up toxins are finally given the boot. The key organs at work here are the liver, lungs, kidneys, skin and digestive system, which act as one to neutralize and transform the toxins we ingest.

Your body has the natural ability to detoxify, but it's easily overburdened by continued exposure to toxic physical and social environments, includ-

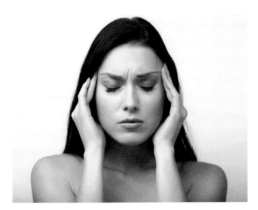

ing pollution, stress, pesticides, food additives, drug residues, poor lifestyle choices and illness. These lead to toxin accumulation, causing fatigue, skin problems, weight gain, mood changes, recurrent infections, insomnia, constipation and other digestive complaints.

What You'll Feel

As your body begins to release built-up toxins you may experience headaches, muscle aches, irritability, nausea, increased urination and/or bowel activity, flu-like symptoms, fatigue and/or skin flare-ups. None of these is life threatening and will not last for long.

Why You'll Feel Like This

If you're feeling this "Hangover," it's likely caused by withdrawal and significant toxin release. Headaches are the result of blood vessel dilation, which is blocked by caffeine. A rebound headache is likely to occur after you cut caffeine from

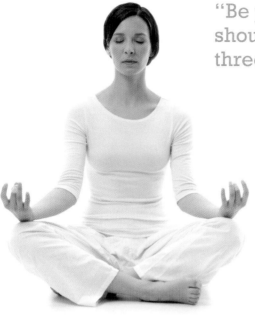

"Be patient. Your symptoms should subside within three to seven days."

10 WAYS TO DEAL WITH THE "CUT THE CRAP" HANGOVER:

1. PRACTICE RELAXATION TECH-NIQUES such as meditation, deep breathing, yoga or tai chi.

2. GET PHYSICAL by working out at a moderate intensity.

3. DRINK PLENTY OF WATER. When you think you've had enough, drink more!

4. INCREASE YOUR FIBER INTAKE MODERATELY (be sure to intake more water, too).

5. DO NOT SKIP MEALS. Eat at regular intervals.

6. GET YOUR VITAMINS AND MINER-ALS by eating a well-balanced diet. You may want to take a multivitamin to ensure you're getting everything your body needs.

7. DRINK NON-CAFFEINATED HERBAL TEAS. Green tea is also beneficial.

8. EAT A BANANA to increase your electrolytes (especially if you've experienced diarrhea).

9. GET A MASSAGE to encourage toxin release.

10. GET PLENTY OF SLEEP – seven to eight hours a night.

your diet. Giving up your addictions to caffeine and sugar will likely cause feelings of withdrawal. Just as toxins build up during exercise, released toxins from organs can accumulate in your muscles, causing tightness and aches, which further aggravates headaches and may cause flu-like symptoms.

When Will the "Cut the Crap" Hangover Go Away?

Be patient. Your symptoms should subside within three to seven days. If your symptoms worsen or continue for more than two weeks, visit your physician. On the other hand, some lucky people never experience detox symptoms at all.

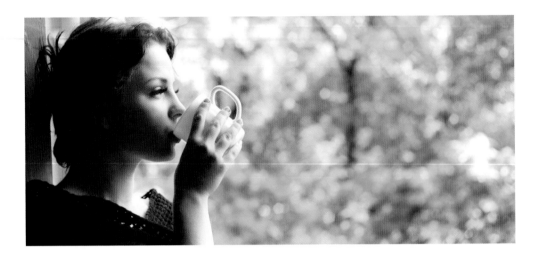

HERBS ARE GREAT FLAVOR-ENHANCERS, but these pleasing plants are known for more than their taste. Herbs have been used for millennia to treat all sorts of digestive disorders, mood problems and stress, to build immunity and fight disease, and some herbs are also used for weight-loss-specific jobs such as helping to control appetite. Some herbs are used rarely for cooking and may be used as a tisane, as an oil or as a tincture. Some examples include St. John's Wort, which helps with mood and depression, chamomile, which helps calm nerves and speeds healing, echinacea, which acts as an immune-system builder, and feverfew, which is a pain reliever.

The following herbs have been shown to assist fat loss through various means including decreasing appetite, increasing metabolism, controlling enzymes, regulating blood sugar or even decreasing cortisol levels, all of which play a role in the process. While I encourage you to add any and all of these plant foods to your diet, you must remember that they work only to aid you in your fat-loss goals – they are not a magic bullet. It seems as soon as a study comes out to support one or another of these substances, suddenly all sorts of people add them to their diet while still gobbling burgers and fries, and then wonder why they aren't losing weight!

You must keep a Clean diet and work out regularly and consistently to lose weight. And if you add these items to your diet you may find the process a little easier. If you are thinking of using any of these foods in supplement form, please discuss with your doctor.

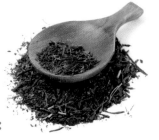

Green Tea:

Green tea is an easy item to add to your daily diet and research has proven it to be effective with weight loss. Green tea helps you burn fat in two ways – through thermogenesis, which raises your metabolism, and through polyphenols, which activate fat-burning enzymes. A few cups of green tea each day (without added sugar, of course!) can help you burn about 70 extra calories.

Spirulina:

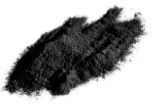

Spirulina was touted as an almost-magic diet food in the 1980s. Of course there is no real magic diet food, but as with the other items on this page it can help in combination with *The Eat-Clean Diet* and an exercise program. Spirulina is blue-green algae, rich in nutrients, which is beneficial to one's health already. When you add in the fact that it helps decrease appetite when consumed before meals, the real magic kicks in.

The jury is out on why spirulina makes people eat less, but most people believe it is spirulina's high protein content in combination with its extremely high nutritional profile. When you consume this superfood, your body recognizes that it does not need as much nutrition from a meal and sends signals to your appetite control center. Whether or not this is the reason, it's an inexpensive food that gives numerous nutritional benefits including a decreased appetite, so it makes sense to include it in your *Stripped* weight-loss plan.

Licorice Root:

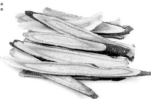

Licorice root in any form helps combat low energy and also helps to keep your bowels moving. When you chew on the actual root itself (which looks like a twig and has a strong licorice flavor), it helps prevent bingeing and satisfies your urge to chew. As a bonus, licorice root can help you quit smoking!

Garcinia Cambogia:

Garcinia cambogia is often seen as a supplement, but it started life as a food. Also known by the names Brindall berries or Malabar tamarind, this food has long been a prized ingredient in foods in certain regions in India. This food has a pleasant sour taste that works well in Asian dishes. The small, pumpkin-like fruit contains hydroxycitric acid, which inhibits the enzyme that helps turn carbohydrates into fat. The theory is that this helps the body burn the extra carbs as energy. Animal studies have shown that this substance not only helps decrease body fat, it also works as an appetite suppressant.

Reishi Mushrooms:

Reishi mushrooms work to lower cortisol levels, and cortisol is that hormone that makes us hold on to fat. Mushrooms in general are a superb food, with anti-cancer and other health properties; reishi mushrooms are some of the most potent. This mushroom also has anti-inflammatory properties and helps those who have problems with anxiety. These mushrooms have a woody texture and are best cooked before eaten.

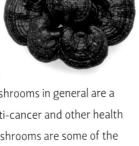

Ginseng:

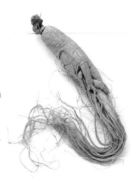

Ginseng, an adaptogen, is commonly used to combat stress, strengthen the immune system and improve health in general. The two most potent and beneficial forms of ginseng are Korean ginseng and American ginseng, and all parts of the plant are used for health purposes, from its roots to its berries. The ginseng root has been used for thousands of years, and is thought to combat many stress-related ailments, balancing hormonal levels and decreasing cortisol overproduction, which also helps with weight control. Recent studies on mice using ginseng berries have found that an extract made from the pulp significantly and positively affected the mice's blood sugar and cholesterol levels in addition to decreasing their appetite and increasing their energy levels. Ginseng can be consumed as a tea or as an extract, but beware when purchasing ginseng products. Ginseng is not inexpensive and many "ginseng" products contain little to no actual ginseng.

> "Ginseng is not inexpensive and many 'ginseng' products contain little to no actual ginseng."

> "Kelp is brown seaweed loaded with vitamins and minerals, including iodine, which helps your thyroid function."

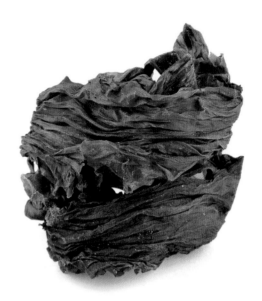

Kelp:

Kelp is brown seaweed loaded with vitamins and minerals, including iodine, which helps your thyroid function. The thyroid gland is the ruler of your metabolism, and you've no doubt heard that those with a sluggish thyroid have decreased energy and gain weight easily. If your thyroid functions well you do not need extra iodine, but some say it can help. Studies on rats show that a substance in kelp, called fucoxanthin, stimulates a protein that helps in the burning of fat.

Holy Basil:

Holy basil, or tulsi, is a common ingredient in Thai food and can also be consumed as a tea. This herb has long been thought to have medicinal qualities, and indeed proves to be a painkiller and adaptogen (which helps combat stress), with strong detoxifying, antibacterial and antioxidant properties. To help with weight loss, holy basil reduces blood glucose and cortisol levels.

Maca:

Maca is a root vegetable grown high in the mountains of central Peru. The root was traditionally used as currency in the area because of its high nutritional value and its reputation for increasing strength and virility. The entire maca plant can be eaten, but most often the term "maca" refers to the root. In its native country the maca root is served many ways, as porridge, as flour or roasted whole for a few examples, but in North America we are most likely to find maca flour, extract or tea. Maca is not only a nutritional powerhouse and an adapotogen helping the body deal with stress, but as an adaptogen it is also a strong hormone regulator – helpful for weight loss. Maca also helps increase energy – another weight-loss aid.

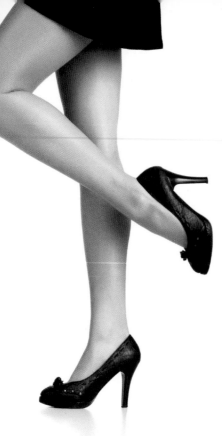

HOW TO LOOK LIKE YOU'VE LOST 10 POUNDS WITHOUT DOING A THING

Sleekify

I talk so much about being your best on the inside, but I don't want you to forget about your outer appearance. I like to leave the house looking my best because it gives me confidence and peace of mind. Plus, when I feel good about myself and the way I look, I'm more likely to follow my *Eat-Clean Diet* plan. These tips will boost your look for a special event or even just to walk to the market to pick up your fruits and veggies – you never know whom you might run into – and they'll help you look leaner, too!

Dressing

We wear clothes every day. Why not select options that make you look slimmer? Stacy and Clinton from TLC's hit show *What Not to Wear* would definitely approve!

> "Wearing heels will make your legs look longer and leaner. They instantly tone up your calves and thighs."

1 Wearing heels will make your legs look longer and leaner.

They instantly tone up your calves and thighs. This is why fitness competitors wear high heels with their suits on stage.

2 Choose clothes that fit.

You may not be in a slim size six yet, but wearing something too small will make you look even bigger! If your waist is a size six but your hips are a size eight, purchase the larger size and have it altered to fit.

3 Trick the eye by choosing clothing with pleasing lines.

V-neck collars make your neck look long and draw attention upward. Slimming A-line skirts will nip in your hips. Accentuating your waist will give you a pleasing hourglass shape. Just be sure to avoid pleats and baggy tops, which will hide what you've been working so hard on.

4 Go monotone with the same color on the top and bottom to look longer and leaner.

5 Choose pants that are long enough.

If your pants are too short, not only will people think you're expecting a flood, but your legs will look much shorter too. Purchase long pants and have them hemmed to the shoes you will wear most often.

6 Wear slimming support wear.

Is there anything more beautiful than the curves of a woman's body? Hold yourself in with support hose, such as Spanx, which can smooth you out from top to bottom. You may struggle to get into them initially, but you will love the finished look. I wear them under those hard-to-hide-a-thing dresses that show every bump.

"Accentuating your waist will give you a pleasing hourglass shape."

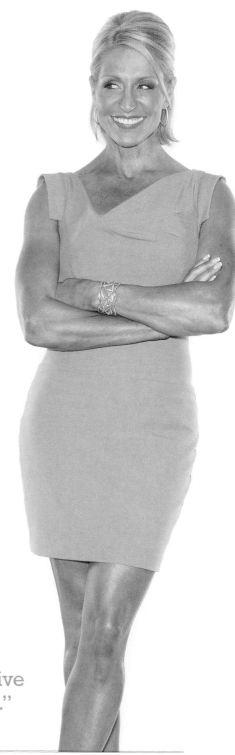

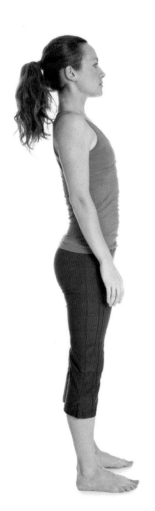

> "If you normally slouch, then you'll appear to lose at least five pounds just by correcting your posture."

Straighten Out

If you normally slouch, then you'll appear to lose at least five pounds just by correcting your posture. Slouching is also hard on your neck muscles, which can lead to headaches. Bad posture causes lower back pain and weak abdominal muscles. Try this: imagine your two hipbones and your pubic bone as the three points of a triangle. Try to keep all three points in line while you are standing to straighten out your lower back. You will feel your abdominal muscles tighten. You can try the same with your shoulder blades. Imagine the points at the base of your shoulder blades shifting down and inwards. This will keep your shoulders back and your chest proud, while preventing tight pectoral muscles and a sore neck.

Get a Glow

Get a spray tan! A body with a bit of color or darkness to it always looks leaner, just as we look leaner wearing darker colors. A tan also helps hide cellulite, a common complaint among women in particular. You may have noticed that it is much more difficult to see cellulite and other flaws on those with darker skin.

Celebs are on to this little nugget, too. Many of the biggest stars like to have a hint of a golden glow to them, because it helps them look tighter and it helps to hide flaws. Stars such as Mariah Carey, Paris Hilton, Lindsay Lohan and Victoria Beckham take full advantage of this trick. Some stars will even hire a specialist who will etch in abs and other muscular definition, along with their healthy glow, to foster the look of fitness.

SUNLESS TANNING

There is no need to spend hours baking yourself in the sun to accomplish your svelte golden glow – that would only speed up

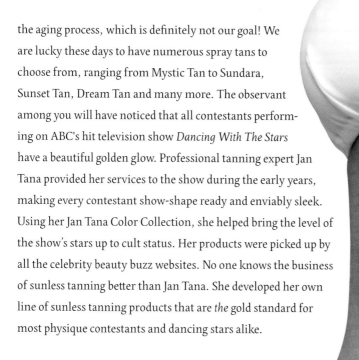

the aging process, which is definitely not our goal! We are lucky these days to have numerous spray tans to choose from, ranging from Mystic Tan to Sundara, Sunset Tan, Dream Tan and many more. The observant among you will have noticed that all contestants performing on ABC's hit television show *Dancing With The Stars* have a beautiful golden glow. Professional tanning expert Jan Tana provided her services to the show during the early years, making every contestant show-shape ready and enviably sleek. Using her Jan Tana Color Collection, she helped bring the level of the show's stars up to cult status. Her products were picked up by all the celebrity beauty buzz websites. No one knows the business of sunless tanning better than Jan Tana. She developed her own line of sunless tanning products that are *the* gold standard for most physique contestants and dancing stars alike.

Plan to get a spray tan at least three days before your debut, whatever the event. I prepare my skin for tanning by giving it a good buffing with exfoliating crystals or an exfoliating mitt – dry skin flakes will make for uneven color. Don't forget to remove unwanted hair in advance of your tan, too. Next, make sure to moisturize your skin so that your spray tan will glide on smoothly. At this point I put on a loosely fitting dark-colored tracksuit with no bra or panties underneath. I let my skin dry thoroughly and then head over to my favorite tanning salon.

If you prefer to apply your own color, make sure to read the product directions carefully. Simply strip off and stand on a

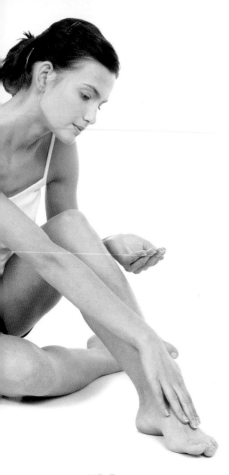

dark towel. Jan Tana always provides a puff with which to apply her color. Apply a few pumps of tan product onto the puff and begin to apply, using long, quick swipes on the body. It doesn't matter where you begin, but be consistent and thorough so you don't miss any spots. I usually do this in front of a mirror so I can see where I am going or if I have missed any bits. Once you have covered your entire body, apply a very light coat on your face. Nothing looks stranger than having a dark body and a white face. Once you are finished, wash out your puff and let it dry. You will also have to let yourself dry, so don't wear any tight-fitting clothing or anything too light in color. I usually throw on a baggy T-shirt and a pair of light, loose cotton pants. Don't exercise or shower for a good six hours. Then give yourself a light, lukewarm rinse in the shower. Don't use soap; just let the water slide off of you – you will see the excess color washing off. Get out and pat dry. Moisturize and enjoy how amazing your new darker color makes you look.

Fix Up Your Face

Eyebrows and cheeks are major accentuating features. Correctly tweezing your brows will instantly liven up your face. Book yourself in for an eyebrow-shaping session at a salon and ask them to put some color and shimmer on your cheeks, too. You will look young and fresh in five minutes flat and you'll have the know-how to do it yourself next time.

Lift the Ladies

Most women wear the wrong size bra, so you might just fall into that category. Most lingerie-store clerks are trained in fitting bras. Go in the week after your period, since breasts tend to swell the week before. Try on different styles until you find a bra that's comfortable and flattering.

> "Most women wear the wrong size bra, so you might just fall into that category."

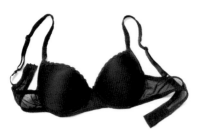

Trim Your Locks

It's amazing how much better a simple change in your hair can make you look. Select a salon and a stylist with a good reputation. Talk to them about the changes you are thinking of making. In just a few hours you'll leave looking years younger.

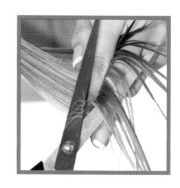

Dazzle Your Dents

A beautiful, white smile can make your face look years younger. Most dentists and dental-hygiene centers offer professional whitening services that don't break the bank. Alternatively, you can use at-home whitening strips, toothpaste and mouthwash to achieve a brighter smile.

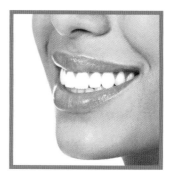

Shimmer

Bring light to the most beautiful parts of your body and face. Shimmer powder can be applied to your cheeks, down the front of your shin, along your shoulder and décolletage. You'll look toned and defined in no time!

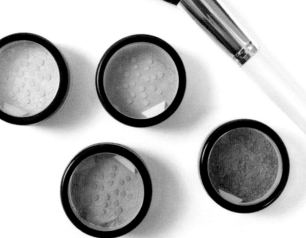

"Bring light
to the most
beautiful parts
of your body
and face."

▶ Cellulite

WHAT IS THAT DIMPLED, ORANGE-PEEL FLESH ON THE BACK OF YOUR LEGS? It's cellulite, and if there ever was an aesthetic reason to slim down, this is it! It tops the list as the least desirable of problems to affect your curves.

What's Going On?

Your skin is composed of layers of connective tissue, including stretchy elastin and tensile collagen. These fibers weave together to create a resilient barrier that serves as your body's first line of defense against foreign objects. Underneath this barrier is a necessary layer of subcutaneous fat, which is important for protection and temperature balance. Unfortunately, a perversion of this fatty layer leads to the appearance of cellulite, or lipodystrophy as it is medically termed. Fat pushes against bands of connective tissue, making the tissue look like unsightly dimpled orange peel. Think of a mattress with its dimpled, quilted outer coating.

There are two types of cellulite - hydric and lipidic. The former is mostly composed of water mixed with a bit of fat, which seeps into tissues and saturates them. The latter tends to collect in localized areas and is predominantly fat. This is the kind that gives the skin the orange-peel appearance often associated with cellulite.

Numerous factors contribute to the development of cellulite including hormones, genetics, lymphatic drainage, diet and exercise. Hormones play a key role in the development of cellulite, which is why it can form during years of maturation in women as they prepare for their childbearing years. As with any other element of your physical being, genetics play a large part in your development. This means if your mom or dad had cellulite you have a greater possibility of developing it too. When damage occurs to the lymphatic system, waste products seep into tissues, accelerating the development of cellulite. Poor diet, especially a lack of protein, will make you more prone to developing cellulite, as will repeated weight gain and loss and insufficient exercise levels. It's your job to alter your nutrition and physical activity levels to avoid developing sloppy, cellulite-ridden flesh.

What to Do:
Procedures, Potions and Perfection:

There is no absolute cure for cellulite, but thanks to today's technology these lumpy bumps can be minimized. A board-certified dermatologist or plastic surgeon can offer a wide range of non-invasive potential cures. Be warned, however, that nothing is guaranteed! Treatments consist of infra-red therapy, as in the popular Vela-Shape procedure, or "cold" lasers, as in the new Zerona.

Going under the knife for corrective surgery is another option, although it is invasive and the possible benefits need to be weighed carefully against other options. There are also numerous creams and lotions claiming to tone, tighten, tuck and more. In combination with massage some of these have been shown mildly effective. They're non-invasive and relatively inexpensive, so give them a try if you wish. Remember that there is no cure for cellulite so your best bet is to avoid developing it in the first place by keeping a Clean diet and active lifestyle. One of my favorite sayings is, "Keep it tight!" And, while I am not an expert, I have noticed that maintaining a "tight" diet keeps cellulite at bay. Don't stray from eating six small meals each day and don't reach for the fake foods that will leave you loathing your lovely legs.

WHAT TO AVOID:

→ **Sugar**

→ **Caffeine**

→ **Smoking**

→ **Excess alcohol**

WHAT TO INCREASE:

Basically any Clean food regimen will enhance your skin and reduce the appearance of cellulite, but certain foods will make the most of your beautiful outer layer. Vitamins, minerals and more are essential to building a healthy, resilient skin layer. Try:

→ **Apples**   → **Beans**

→ **Eggs**   → **Fish**

→ **Nuts**   → **Asparagus**

WHEN TO EXPECT RESULTS:

In as little as three weeks you will notice your skin glowing and looking brighter as it reestablishes its suppleness, resilience and luster. Eating properly is the surest and least expensive approach to achieving healthy skin and most of all maintaining it! It is as simple as making small changes towards selecting healthier foods – that is what the Eat-Clean lifestyle is all about.

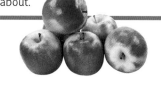

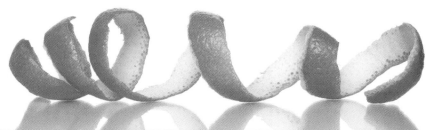

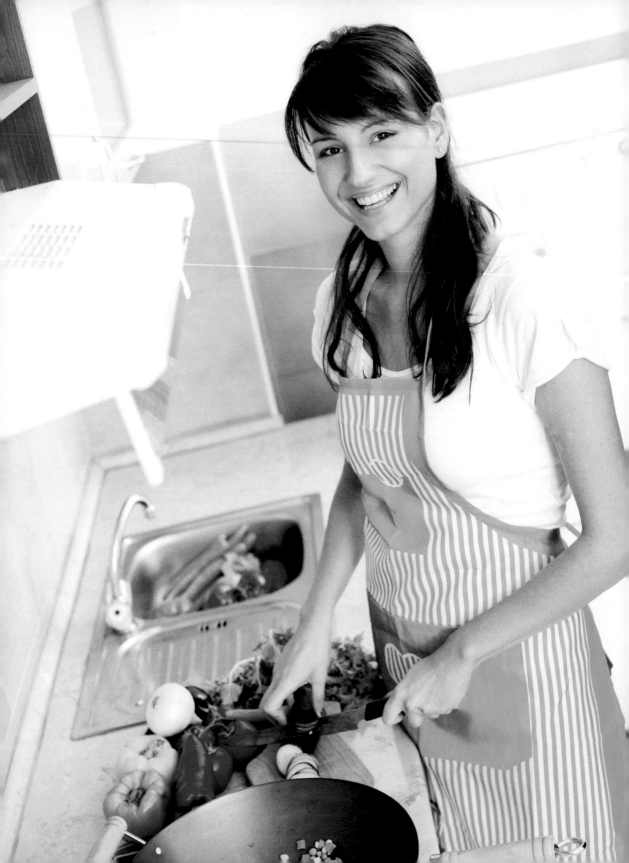

11 | Meal Plans

This chapter will be your go-to guide throughout your *Stripped* journey. This is your overview of the next 28 days: you'll find the *Stripped* Cooler plan, the *Eat-Clean Diet* Principles, portion-size guidelines and two weeks of meal plans to get you started on defeating those last 10 pounds. After you've got all the essentials, turn the page to find a condensed version of the *Stripped* plan. This info sheet includes tips on which foods to choose, how much water to drink and even advice for speeding up your weight loss. Get familiar with *The Eat-Clean Diet Stripped* in just one glance – the slim, toned body of your dreams is just four weeks away!

Your *Stripped* Cooler Plan Explained

Your *Stripped* Cooler Plan is meant for four weeks' worth of food. This plan, along with regular workouts including cardio and strength training, will help you lose those last 10 pounds.

Read over the Eat-Clean Principles on page 54 and refer to this checklist when packing your daily cooler.

1. Eat more! Eat six small meals each day, spaced at two-and-a-half to three-hour intervals.

2. Eat breakfast every day, within an hour of rising.

3. Make your last meal three hours before bed.

4. Eat a combination of lean protein and complex carbohydrates at each meal.

5. Eat sufficient healthy fats every day.

6. Drink two to three liters of water each day.

7. Carry a cooler packed with Clean foods each day.

8. Depend on fresh fruits and vegetables for fiber, vitamins, nutrients and enzymes.

9. Adhere to proper portion sizes.

10. Eat only foods that have not been overly processed or doused in chemicals, saturated and trans fats and/or toxins.

YOUR *STRIPPED* COOLER PLAN: PEEL OFF THOSE LAST 10 POUNDS

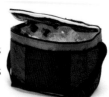

What It's for:

* Losing those last 10 pounds
* Preparing for special events
* Boosting self-esteem
* Improving your health
* Showing increased muscular definition

What It Is:

The *Stripped* Cooler Plan is a four-week-long plan to help you lose those last 10 pounds and get in your best shape ever. It's a restrictive plan yet you won't feel overly hungry because you'll be eating a combination of foods that fill you up and give you abundant energy to get through your busy day, while blasting fat at the same time.

How It Works:

Abide by the menu plans that begin on page 190. Follow the two-week plan as written, then repeat it for the following two weeks. Your four weeks will look like this:

Week 1: Week 1 Menu Plan

Week 2: Week 2 Menu Plan

Week 3: Week 1 Menu Plan

Week 4: Week 2 Menu Plan

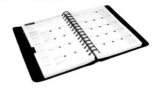

Portion-Size Guidelines

Lean Protein:

One palm-sized portion at each meal.

ALLOWABLE FOODS: egg whites, lean turkey and chicken breast, lean pork, beans and legumes (in moderation), lean fish (tuna, salmon, trout, cod, halibut, etc.), shrimp, clams, mussels, bison and other game meats, hummus (also a healthy fat), quinoa, spirulina, sea vegetables, protein powder, tofu and tempeh.

Starchy Complex Carbohydrates:

One or two cupped handfuls per day, divided between one or two meals.

ALLOWABLE FOODS: sweet potatoes, potatoes, radishes, beans and legumes (also a protein), oats, brown rice, bananas, carrots, parsnips, bulgur wheat, teff and farro.

Complex Carbohydrates from Fruits and Vegetables:

Two cupped handfuls at each meal.

ALLOWABLE FOODS: apples, plums, berries, pears, tomatoes, cucumber, broccoli, asparagus, beets, leeks, spinach and other leafy greens (the darker the better), Brussels sprouts, green beans, onions, sprouts, celery, watermelon, cherries, zucchini, fennel, oranges, limes, lemons and garlic.

Healthy Fats:

One to two servings per day, divided between one or two meals.

ALLOWABLE FOODS: Flaxseed, nuts (almonds, walnuts and pumpkin seeds are best in moderation), natural nut butters, hummus (also a protein), avocados, oils (sesame, coconut, olive, hazelnut, walnut and fish).

OTHER ALLOWABLE FOODS: Coffee, caffeine-free herbal tea, tamari, unsweetened soy, rice or almond milk, mustard, salsa, herbs and spices.

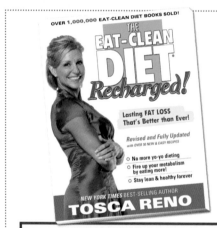

NOTE: If you have more than 10 pounds to lose, or if you have met your weight-loss goals and want to maintain your weight, follow my Cooler 2 Plan, found in *The Eat-Clean Diet Recharged!* It is the plan I follow every day!

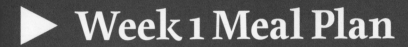

▶ Week 1 Meal Plan

	BREAKFAST BOOSTER	MIDMORNING MUNCH	LUNCHTIME REFUEL
MON	Be A Master of Your Frittata (pg. 205); black coffee; water	Handful of almonds; 1 apple; water	Baked chicken breast sliced onto raw spinach with chopped onion & tomato, black beans & a squeeze of lemon; water
TUE	Oatmeal with chopped apple & cinnamon; 4 egg whites, scrambled; black coffee; water	Go Green Smoothie (pg. 217); water	Light and Lean Leek and Potato Soup (pg. 222); grilled chicken breast; water
WED	Take Me On Vacation Oatmeal (pg. 210); black coffee; water	2 hard-boiled eggs; berries; water	Ladies' Lunch Quick Shrimp Ceviche Stuffed Avocados (pg. 234); water
THU	Oatmeal with ½ banana, sliced; chopped walnuts; 4 hard-boiled egg whites; black coffee; water	½ chicken breast; steamed green beans; water	Leftover bison tenderloin sliced over raw spinach with sliced radishes, strawberries & chopped almonds; squeeze of lemon juice; water
FRI	Protein smoothie: 2 plums, oats, lemon juice, water, vanilla protein powder, ice cubes & unsweetened almond milk; black coffee; water	1 apple; water-packed canned tuna; water	Easy Emerald City Bouillabaisse (pg. 225); water
SAT	Cooked quinoa topped with unsweetened almond milk, blueberries, raspberries & cinnamon; black coffee; water	Strawberries; 1 handful cashews; water	1 leftover salmon dinner; water
SUN	Rise 'n' Shine Teff Grain Breakfast Bowl (pg. 202); black coffee; water	Protein shake: 1 scoop protein powder, water; 1 pear; water	Leftover tilapia dinner; water

MID-AFTERNOON PICK-ME-UP	DINNERTIME DELIGHT	BEFORE BED (if hungry)
2 hard-boiled eggs; celery; water	Roasted turkey breast; steamed broccoli; brown rice; water	4 scrambled egg whites with sliced tomato; caffeine-free herbal tea
Strawberries; 1 handful cashews; water	Backyard BBQ Broccolini (pg. 250); baked trout; brown rice; water	1 apple; protein shake: 1 scoop protein powder, water; caffeine-free herbal tea
1 pear; water-packed canned tuna; water	Bison tenderloin; roasted carrots, beets, leeks & sweet potatoes; water	Handful of almonds; 1 apple; caffeine-free herbal tea
Protein shake: 1 scoop protein powder, water; 1 pear	Lots o' Peppers Seafood and Black Bean Chili (pg. 230); water	4 scrambled egg whites with sliced tomato; caffeine-free herbal tea
Chopped apple, pear & blueberries topped with chopped walnuts & a squeeze of lemon juice; water	Salmon with Sweet 'n' Tangy Pineapple Chutney (pg. 282); brown rice; Sassy Southern Greens (pg. 241); water	1 sliced apple spread with almond butter; caffeine-free herbal tea
Hummus with sliced cucumber; water	Baked tilapia; steamed spinach; sliced tomatoes; water	Small serving of leftover breakfast; caffeine-free herbal tea
Chopped apple, pear & blueberries topped with chopped walnuts and a squeeze of lemon juice; water	Not Your Mom's Elk Pot Roast with Root Vegetable Sauce (pg. 281); water	Protein shake: 1 scoop protein powder, water; banana; caffeine-free herbal tea

Week 2 Meal Plan

	BREAKFAST BOOSTER	MIDMORNING MUNCH	LUNCHTIME REFUEL
MON	Oatmeal topped with blueberries, strawberries & chopped walnuts; 4 egg whites scrambled; black coffee; water	1 apple; water-packed canned tuna; water	Baked chicken breast sliced onto raw spinach with chopped onion & tomato, black beans & a squeeze of lemon; water
TUE	Rise 'n' Shine Teff Grain Breakfast Bowl (pg. 202); black coffee; water	Hummus; red pepper slices; water	Sweetheart Shrimp and Watermelon Salad (pg. 238); water
WED	Oatmeal with chopped apple & cinnamon; 4 egg whites, scrambled; black coffee; water	2 celery stalks topped with almond butter; water	Leftover salmon dinner; water
THU	Protein smoothie: almond milk, protein powder, flaxseed, blueberries, 1 banana & ice cubes; black coffee; water	2 hard-boiled eggs; Keep It Cool Cucumber Melon Ice Pops (pg. 221); water	Tasty Naked Wonton Soup (pg. 226); water
FRI	Take Me On Vacation Oatmeal (pg. 210); black coffee; water	2 hard-boiled eggs; 1 pear; water	Canned, water-packed tuna over romaine lettuce with sprouts & a squirt of lemon juice; water
SAT	Cooked quinoa topped with unsweetened almond milk, blueberries, raspberries & cinnamon; black coffee; water	Mixed nuts and seeds; berries; water	Leftover quinoa, tomatoes, cucumbers tossed with balsamic vinegar & olive oil; water
SUN	Be A Master of Your Frittata (pg. 205); black coffee; water	Chopped apple, pear & blueberries topped with chopped walnuts and a squeeze of lemon juice; water	Scallops a la Plancha with Sautéed Asparagus and Peppers (pg. 269); water

For a sample *Stripped* grocery list, visit: **www.eatcleandiet.com/strippedgrocerylist**

MID-AFTERNOON PICK-ME-UP	DINNERTIME DELIGHT	BEFORE BED (if hungry)
2 hard-boiled eggs; 1 banana; water	Chinese Five Spice Venison with Indian Eggplant (pg. 277); water	4 scrambled egg whites with sliced tomato; caffeine-free herbal tea
Protein shake: 1 scoop protein powder, water; 1 pear	Baked salmon; baked sweet potato; roasted Brussels sprouts; water	Small chicken breast; sliced cucumber; caffeine-free herbal tea
½ chicken breast; 1 sliced tomato; water	Baked chicken breast; steamed green beans & zucchini; brown rice; water	Strawberries; 1 handful cashews; caffeine-free herbal tea
Handful of almonds; 1 apple; water	When the Weather is Frightful, Make Delightful Roasted Butternut Squash Farro Risotto (pg. 262); water	4 scrambled egg whites with sliced tomato; caffeine-free herbal tea
Strawberries; 1 handful cashews; water	Baked trout; Vegetables à la Grecque (pg. 246); brown rice; water	1 sliced apple spread with almond butter; caffeine-free herbal tea
Hummus with sliced cucumber; water	Bison tenderloin; roasted beets, leeks & Brussels sprouts; water	Protein shake: 1 scoop protein powder, water; 1 pear; caffeine-free herbal tea
1 apple; water-packed canned tuna; water	Stir-Fried Ginger Beef with Snap Peas, Shiitake Mushrooms and Red Peppers (pg. 278); water	Hummus; cherry tomatoes; caffeine-free herbal tea

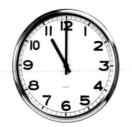

The Eat-Clean Diet *Stripped* At a Glance

An at-a-glance info sheet for losing those last 10 stubborn pounds in four weeks fast! This condensed version of *The Eat-Clean Diet Stripped* provides a glimpse of what you can expect as you tackle losing those sticky remaining 10 pounds. This is a four-week plan to slim and tone yourself into the shape of your dreams.

How many meals will I be able to eat?

You will eat five to six meals per day. Starting with breakfast in the morning as your first meal, all other meals will be eaten at two-and-a-half to three-hour intervals until your last meal has been consumed.

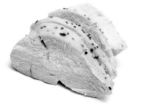

What will those meals look like?

Following the *Stripped* meal plan means you will eat appropriately sized meals using your hands as a guide for measuring portion size (see page 64 for more on portion sizes). You will not be starving yourself to accomplish weight loss.

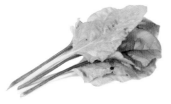

What sort of foods will I eat?

The backbone of *The Eat-Clean Diet* involves partnering lean protein with complex carbohydrates at each meal. This combination of nutrients has been proven to maintain steady blood-glucose levels and prolong digestion so you feel full and satisfied longer. These foods also stimulate your own fat burning mechanism – your metabolism. There will be no calorie counting, so you can breathe a sigh of relief! Your *Stripped* meal plan also advocates eating enough healthy fats, which will actually stimulate fat burning.

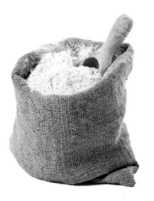

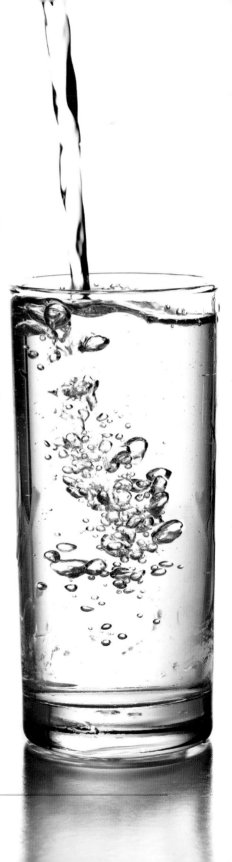

What should I avoid?

You should avoid all over-processed, chemically charged, toxin-laden foods. Sugar in all its disguises and white refined flour products are at the top of the list of no-no foods. Let me add here that alcohol is just another form of sugar so it is critical to avoid alcohol during your four-week plan. Your success will depend on it. It is also important to stay away from unhealthy fats and foods containing excess sodium. In general, if you don't recognize the ingredients don't eat the food.

What should I eat a lot of?

There are several foods that you will be eating a lot of during the next four weeks. These include egg whites, lean turkey and chicken breasts, nuts, berries, beans and legumes, spinach and other leafy greens, green vegetables (especially beans), asparagus and broccoli, bison, pumpkin and sweet potatoes, oats, quinoa and apples.

How much water should I drink?

Your Eat-Clean beverage of choice is water and you should drink at least two to three liters per day, more if you are physically active (which you should be!). You can also drink black coffee and as much caffeine-free herbal tea as you like. Remember: no sugar – not even fakes or alternatives, and no milk!

"Your Eat-Clean beverage of choice is water and you should drink at least two to three liters per day, more if you are physically active."

TOSCA'S PROTEIN SMOOTHIE

1 serving
2 cups / 480 ml per serving

INGREDIENTS

1 cup / 240 ml fresh or frozen
  mixed berries
1 cup / 240 ml unflavored rice milk
2 Tbsp / 30 ml flaxseed
1 scoop protein powder

METHOD

Blend all ingredients and drink.

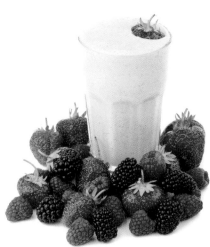

▲ **SHORT ON TIME?** A protein smoothie is the perfect go-to meal in a glass.

I need a go-to Eat-Clean meal. What do you suggest?

Having a quick go-to meal at the ready to stave off hunger and possible binge eating is your secret weapon in the *Stripped* four-week plan. Using a good-quality protein powder (see protein powder reference guide on page 140), know how to whip up a protein- and nutrient-rich smoothie in minutes so you stay satisfied and healthy. My ideal meal recipe is to the left.

Do I have to work out?

Yes, workouts are a must! The best way to accelerate the loss of those final 10 pounds is to include regular workouts as part of your weight-loss regimen. You will work out six times per week, alternating cardio training with weight training, and your seventh day is for rest. Resistance training with weights is an important part of your *Stripped* plan. When you build lean muscle you increase your metabolic rate and your fat-burning speed.

How can I speed up my weight loss?

You've got to train the big guns! This is another secret of your *Stripped* plan. When you train the largest muscle groups in your body you will over-stimulate your metabolism, pushing it into overdrive. In so doing you will accelerate the regular rate of fat burning way beyond its normal capacity. The more you train these large muscle groups the better – so target your glutes and quads frequently!

"You will work out six times per week, alternating cardio training with weight training, and your seventh day is for rest. "

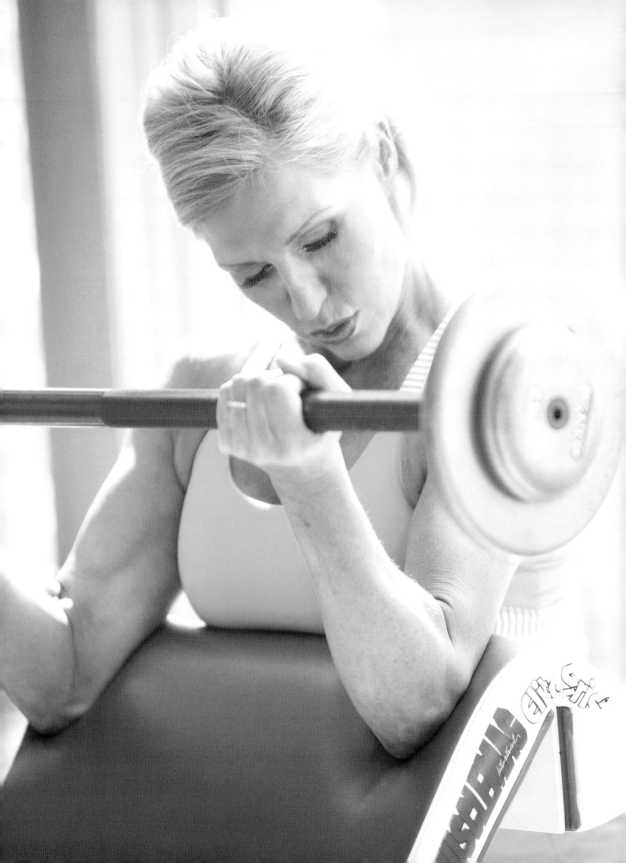

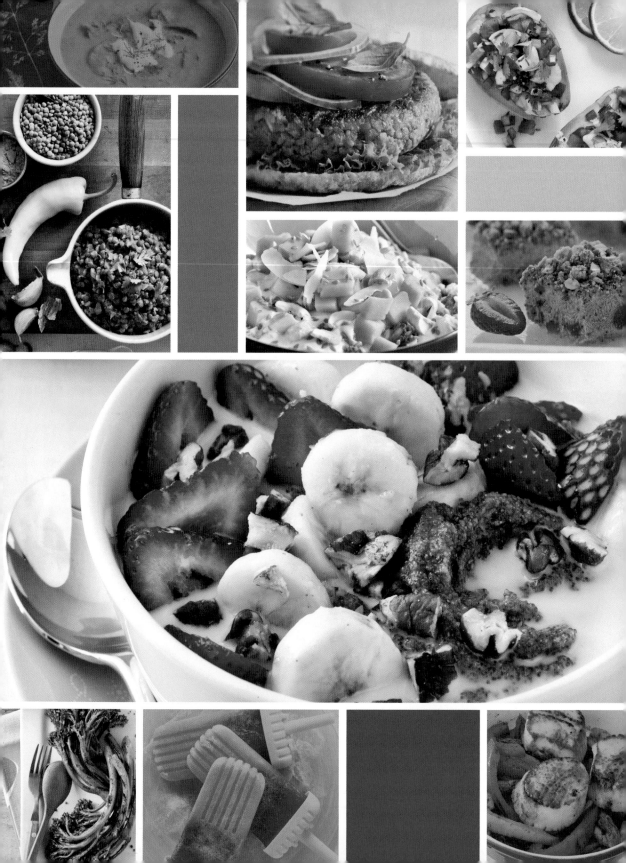

12 | Stripped Recipes

hether you're looking for a meal for one or something savory to share, we've got your *Stripped* menus covered! Here you'll find 52 brand new recipes to jump-start your metabolism and keep it burning all day. Start your morning right with the Rise 'n' Shine Teff Grain Breakfast Bowl, satisfy your sweet tooth with the Strawberry Dreamboat Bars or share a cozy evening with your special someone with the My Heart Sings for You Halibut for Two. Best of all, you'll be able to stick to your *Stripped* plan easily with these scrumptious, good-for-you recipes that are chock full of vital nutrients and bursting with flavor. Bon appétit!

TABLE OF CONTENTS

FAMILY-FRIENDLY RECIPES

These recipes contain grain products making them a family-friendly option. Omit the grain products if you are following the *Eat-Clean Diet Stripped* plan.

TREATS

These recipes are treats and should not be consumed when following the *Eat-Clean Diet Stripped* plan. They can be reintroduced into your weekly menus once you reach your maintenance period.

Rise 'n' Shine Teff Grain Breakfast Bowl

2 servings
(1½ cups / 360 ml per serving)

PREP: 2 minutes

TOTAL: 19 minutes

Teff is a tiny cereal grain that has been popular in Northern Africa for centuries. The word "teff" means "lost," a reference to the size of the grain. It's so small that if dropped, it's impossible to find! However, you can find it at a health food store or large grocery market.

Ingredients

¼ cup / 60 ml whole grain teff

Scant pinch sea salt

1 tsp / 5 ml flaxseed meal or ground flaxseed

¼ tsp / 1.25 ml ground cinnamon

½ cup / 120 ml unsweetened almond milk

1 small banana, or ½ large, sliced

1 cup / 240 ml sliced strawberries

2 Tbsp / 30 ml pecan pieces

Nutritional Value Per Serving:

Calories: 275 | Calories from Fat: 103 |
Protein: 7 g | Carbs: 40 g |
Total Fat: 11 g | Saturated Fat: 1 g |
Trans Fat: 0 g | Fiber: 7 g |
Sodium: 212 mg | Cholesterol: 0 mg |
Sugar: 11 g

Method

1   In a small saucepan, bring 1 cup / 240 ml of water to boil. Add teff and pinch of sea salt, cover and simmer until the water is absorbed, stirring occasionally, 15 minutes. Remove from heat, stir and let sit, covered, for three minutes.

2   Stir in flax and cinnamon. Divide equally between two bowls; pour almond milk over teff and top with banana, strawberries and pecans.

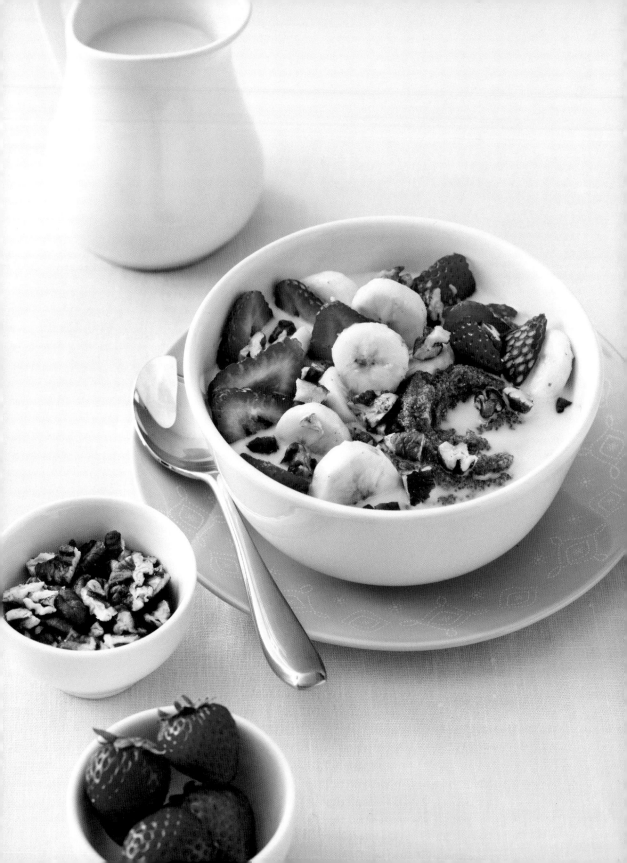

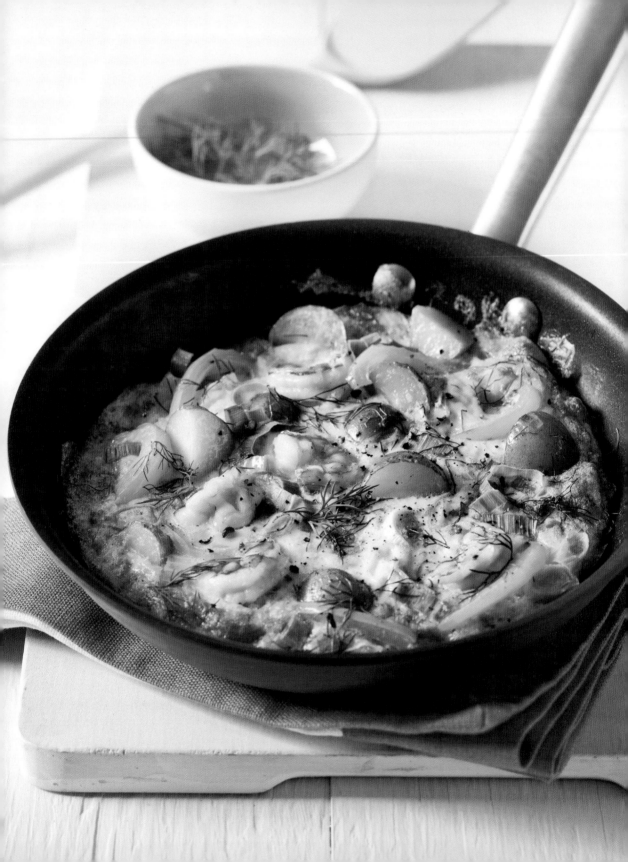

Be a Master of Your Frittata

2 servings

PREP: 10 minutes

TOTAL: 15 to 17 minutes

Frittatas are quick to prepare and a great choice for breakfast, dinner and even tomorrow's lunch. Take a "kitchen sink" approach to making your frittata. Experiment with different ingredients (try raw veggies and yesterday's leftovers) until you find the perfect combination for your palate.

Ingredients

BASE:
1 egg

5 egg whites

¼ tsp / 1.25 ml sea salt

⅛ tsp / pinch freshly ground black pepper

Eat-Clean Cooking Spray (see page 214 for recipe)

FRITTATA:
Choose ¾ cup / 180 ml to 1 cup / 240 ml each of vegetables, protein and starches/grains):

Vegetables:
Asparagus, raw or cooked

Bell peppers, raw or cooked

Chili peppers, raw or cooked

Greens (arugula, kale, mustard, spinach), raw or cooked

Leeks, raw or cooked

Mushrooms (any kind), raw or cooked

Scallions, raw or cooked

Yellow squash, raw or cooked

Zucchini, raw or cooked

Proteins:
Bay shrimp, cooked

Prawns, cooked

Chicken breast, cooked

Lean pork, cooked

Salmon, cooked

Trout, cooked

Starches and Grains:
Potatoes (baby red, Yukon gold or russet), cooked

Quinoa, cooked

Brown rice, cooked

Choose 1 tsp / 5 ml of chopped fresh herbs:

Basil

Chives

Cilantro

Dill

Parsley

Tarragon

Nutritional Value Per Serving ✱ :

Calories: 127 | Calories from Fat: 30 | Protein: 17 g | Carbs: 7 g | Total Fat: 2.75 g | Saturated Fat: 1 g | Trans Fat: 0 g | Fiber: 0.9 g | Sodium: 418 mg | Cholesterol: 113.5 mg | Sugar: 1 g

✱ NI for frittata with ¼ cup / 60 ml chopped bell peppers, ¼ cup / 60 ml chopped mushrooms, ¼ / 60 ml cup chopped chicken breast and ¼ cup / 60 ml cooked brown rice.

Method

1 Move rack in oven to second highest position. Preheat oven to broil.

2 Whisk together frittata base ingredients except Eat-Clean Cooking Spray. Chop selected vegetables into one-inch pieces. Chop precooked proteins and potatoes into one-inch pieces. Chop herbs if using.

3 Heat an eight-inch nonstick, oven-safe sauté pan over medium heat and coat with Cooking Spray. Add vegetables to pan and sauté for two minutes until they start to soften. Add remaining ingredients (proteins, starches/grains) then pour egg mixture into pan. Sprinkle in herb of choice and stir with rubber spatula. Cook for two to three minutes, or until egg mixture is set on bottom and beginning to set on top.

4 Place pan into oven and broil for two minutes, until lightly browned and fluffy. Remove frittata from pan and cut into four wedges.

Gold Medal Finish Breakfast Burrito (Ⓜ)

2 servings

PREP: 10 minutes

TOTAL: 20 minutes

This breakfast burrito means serious business. It's hearty enough to take you to your next meal and power you through – or refuel you after – an intense workout. Try it tomorrow morning or any time of day!

Ingredients

Eat-Clean Cooking Spray (see page 214 for recipe)

6 oz / 170 g extra lean ground turkey

1 tsp / 5 ml ground cumin

¼ tsp / 1.25 ml garlic powder

4 egg whites

¼ tsp / 1.25 ml sea salt

⅛ tsp / pinch freshly ground black pepper

⅓ cup / 80 ml drained and rinsed black beans

⅓ cup / 80 ml drained and chopped roasted red peppers

2 cups / 480 ml lightly packed fresh spinach

¼ cup / 60 ml hummus, homemade or store bought

2 whole grain sprouted tortillas (such as Ezekiel), warmed (optional)

Chipotle Mexican hot sauce, to taste (optional)

Note: Skip the tortilla if you are following the *Stripped* plan.

Nutritional Value Per Serving:

Calories: 351 | Calories from Fat: 91 | Protein: 32 g | Carbs: 30 g | Total Fat: 8 g | Saturated Fat: 1.8 g | Trans Fat: 0 g | Fiber: 8 g | Sodium: 988 mg | Cholesterol: 42 mg | Sugar: 2 g

Method

1 Heat a large nonstick skillet over medium-high heat, and if necessary, spray with Eat-Clean Cooking Spray. Add ground turkey, cumin and garlic powder, and use a wooden spatula to break the meat into small pieces. Cook until no longer pink, two minutes.

2 Add egg whites to same skillet, season mixture with salt and pepper, and stir until opaque, two minutes. Add black beans, roasted red peppers and spinach, and stir all ingredients together.

3 Spread hummus on warm tortillas (skip if you are following the *Stripped* plan), then top with turkey mixture and top with chipotle hot sauce, if desired. Roll up burritos and eat warm.

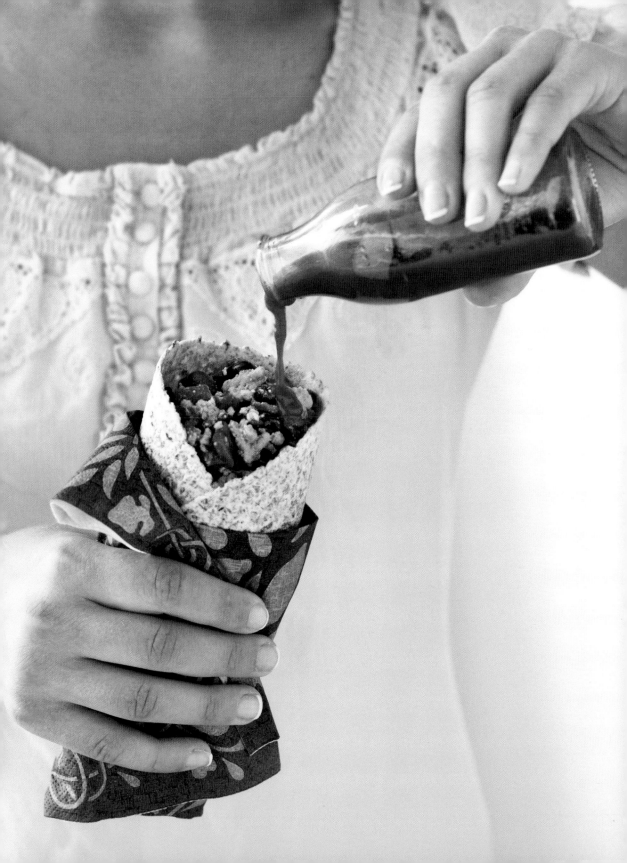

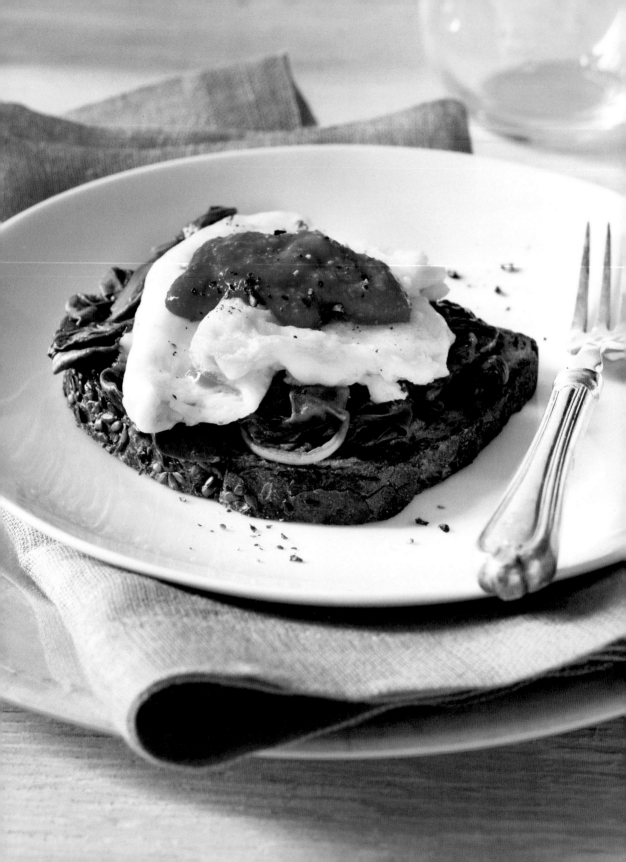

Weekend Brunch Eggs Florentine on Hearty Rye with Romesco ⊛

2 servings

PREP: 15 minutes

TOTAL: 115 minutes

Romesco is a rich sauce from the Catalan region of Spain. It's called a sauce, but it's more like a sidedish, dip or chutney with a powerful flavor. This recipe yields about a cup, so you'll have leftovers to use on top of grilled vegetables, egg-white omelets, whole grains or fish.

Note: Skip the bread if you are following the *Stripped* plan.

Nutritional Value Per Serving (1 slice toast, half of wilted spinach, 2 egg whites, 2 to 3 Tbsp / 30 to 45 ml Romesco):

Calories: 251 | Calories from Fat: 91 | Protein: 18 g | Carbs: 28 g | Total Fat: 10.5 g | Saturated Fat: 1.3 g | Trans Fat: 0 g | Fiber: 8 g | Sodium: 845 mg | Cholesterol: 0 mg | Sugar: 6 g

Ingredients

ROMESCO:

2 tomatoes, cores removed

1 head garlic

2 tsp / 10 ml olive oil, divided

2 Tbsp / 30 ml almond slices or slivers

½ cup / 120 ml jarred roasted red bell peppers, drained

1 tsp / 5 ml red wine vinegar

½ tsp / 2.5 ml sea salt

¼ tsp / 1.25 ml freshly ground black pepper

EGGS FLORENTINE:

4 cups / 960 ml baby spinach, packed

Eat-Clean Cooking Spray (see page 214 for recipe)

4 egg whites

Sea salt and freshly ground black pepper

2 slices hearty whole grain rye bread, toasted (optional)

Method

ROMESCO:

1 Preheat oven to 375°F / 190°C. Place tomatoes on a baking sheet. Cut off top third of garlic and discard. Place remaining garlic head in a piece of aluminum foil and place on baking sheet with tomatoes. Drizzle 1 tsp / 5 ml olive oil into cored tomato wells and on top of garlic. Bring ends of foil together around garlic and squeeze shut. Place baking sheet in oven and roast until garlic and tomatoes are caramelized, but not burnt, one to one-and-a-half hours. Remove and set aside to cool.

2 While tomatoes and garlic are cooling, place almonds on a baking sheet and toast in oven until lightly browned, about five minutes. Remove and set aside to cool.

3 Squeeze half of roasted garlic cloves out of bulb into a food processor and add tomatoes. Add 1 tsp / 5 ml olive oil, almonds, vinegar, salt and pepper, and blend until very smooth, stopping processor once or twice to scrape down sides. Remove to a bowl and set aside. Store leftover garlic in refrigerator.

EGGS FLORENTINE:

1 Heat a large nonstick pan over medium heat. Add spinach and using tongs, fold spinach over a few times to wilt. Remove from heat and set aside.

2 Heat a small- to medium-sized nonstick pan over medium-low heat and spray with Eat-Clean Cooking Spray. Add two egg whites, and let spread out evenly. When almost set, sprinkle with a pinch of salt and pepper, and, using a rubber spatula, fold over edges into the shape of a square. Remove and set aside. Repeat with remaining two egg whites.

3 Top each piece of toasted rye (skip if you are following the *Stripped* plan) with spinach, cooked egg whites and 2 to 3 Tbsp / 30 to 45 ml Romesco.

Take Me On Vacation Oatmeal

2 servings
(1½ cups per serving)

PREP: 15 minutes

TOTAL: 10 minutes

There are so many ways to liven up the dishes you eat on a daily basis. This oatmeal is just one example of a recipe that's healthy, hearty and anything but boring! The pairing of coconut and mango makes you feel like you're miles away, and the addition of protein powder makes it a complete Clean meal.

Ingredients

½ cup / 120 ml old-fashioned rolled oats (not instant)

½ cup / 120 ml oat bran

⅛ tsp / pinch sea salt

1 cup / 240 ml unsweetened almond milk

¼ cup / 60 ml protein powder (optional)

1 ripe mango, peeled and pitted, diced

1 tsp / 5 ml roasted golden flaxseed

2 Tbsp / 30 ml chopped cashews

1 Tbsp / 15 ml unsweetened flaked coconut

Nutritional Value Per Serving:

Calories: 317 | Calories from Fat: 108 | Protein: 10.5 g | Carbs: 53 g | Total Fat: 13 g | Saturated Fat: 3 g | Trans Fat: 0 g | Fiber: 9 g | Sodium: 193 mg | Cholesterol: 0 mg | Sugar: 17 g

Method

1 Combine oats, oat bran and salt with 2¼ cups / 540 ml water in a small saucepan over medium-high heat until simmering. Reduce heat to low and cook, stirring, until mixture thickens and water is absorbed, about three minutes. Remove from heat and let sit two minutes.

2 Divide cereal equally between two bowls. Whisk together almond milk and protein powder, and pour over cereal. Top with mango, flaxseed, cashews and coconut.

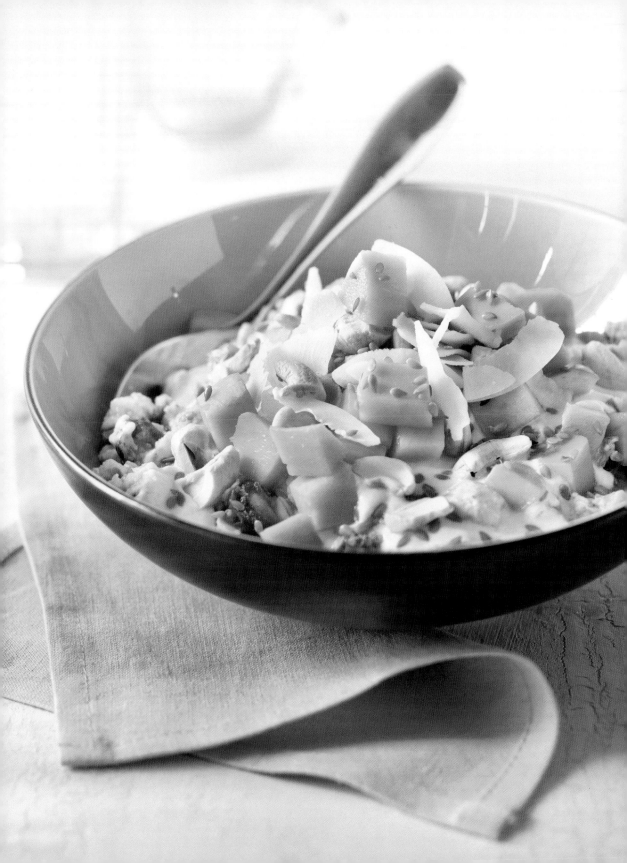

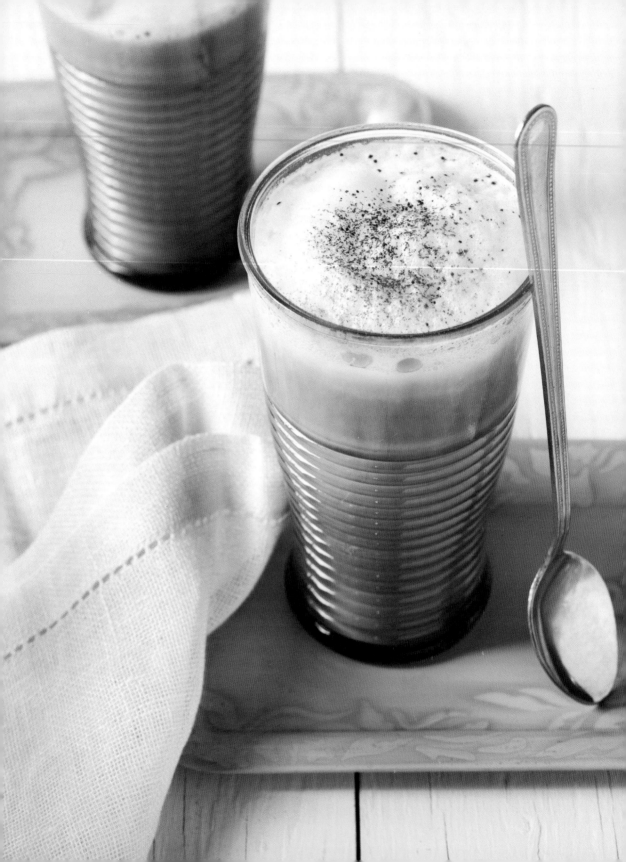

Skinny Soy Mocha

After you try this delicous low-fat soy latte, you'll never waste your hard-earned dollars at the overpriced coffee shop again! Don't like soy? Try it with rice, almond or oat milk.

Ingredients

3 Tbsp / 45 ml freshly ground
espresso roast coffee

1 Tbsp + ¼ tsp / 15 ml + 1.25 ml
cocoa powder, divided

½ cup / 120 ml plain unsweetened
soy milk

¼ tsp / 1.25 ml real vanilla extract

Nutritional Value Per Serving:

Calories: 70 | Calories from Fat: 8 |
Protein: 5 g | Carbs: 8 g | Total Fat: 3 g |
Saturated Fat: 0 g | Trans Fat: 0 g |
Fiber: 3 g | Sodium: 67 mg |
Cholesterol: 0 mg | Sugar: 3 g

Method

1   Add coffee and 1 Tbsp / 15 ml cocoa powder to a lined single-cup coffee filter, such as a Melitta (you could also use a French press to brew coffee). Add 1 cup / 240 ml boiling water and allow to pass through filter into a coffee mug underneath.

2   In a small saucepan, add soy milk, remaining cocoa powder and vanilla extract. Heat milk mixture over medium-high heat while whisking vigorously (use those arm muscles!) until cocoa powder is dissolved and milk is hot and foamy.

3   Pour milk mixture into coffee mug, reserving some foam to place on top. Dust with a little more cocoa powder, if desired, and drink immediately.

Chili Cheese Popcorn 🎎

2 servings
(2 cups / 480 ml per serving)

PREP: 5 minutes

TOTAL: 5 minutes

Eating Clean does not mean depriving yourself. You can eat your old favorites, such as popcorn, so long as you Clean it up a little. This recipe calls for nutritional yeast, an inactive yeast that's popular with vegans. It's got a nutty, cheesy taste and it's also high in vitamin B12, so you can feel good about your choice of movie munchie. This is a treat that should only be enjoyed twice at most on your *Stripped* program.

Ingredients

¼ cup / 60 ml popcorn kernels

Eat-Clean Cooking Spray
   (recipe below)

½ tsp / 2.5 ml chili powder

2 tsp / 10 ml nutritional yeast

¼ tsp / 1.25 ml sea salt

Nutritional Value Per Serving:

Calories: 58 | Calories from Fat: 8 | Protein: 1.7 g | Carbs: 11 g | Total Fat: 0.6 g | Saturated Fat: 0 g | Trans Fat: 0 g | Fiber: 2.5 g | Sodium: 242 mg | Cholesterol: 0 mg | Sugar: 0 g

Method

1 Using an air popper, pop popcorn.

2 Spray popped corn with Eat-Clean Cooking Spray, enough to moisten kernels and allow ingredients to stick. Sprinkle with chili powder, nutritional yeast and salt. Toss to combine.

Eat-Clean Cooking Spray

Cooking sprays such as Pam and others are very handy, but I have become concerned about the presence of isobutane as an ingredient. My solution is to put healthy oils such as extra virgin olive oil inside a spritz bottle, and simply spritz my pans and baking sheets when ready to use. Voilà! Healthy Eat-Clean Cooking Spray with no questionable ingredients.

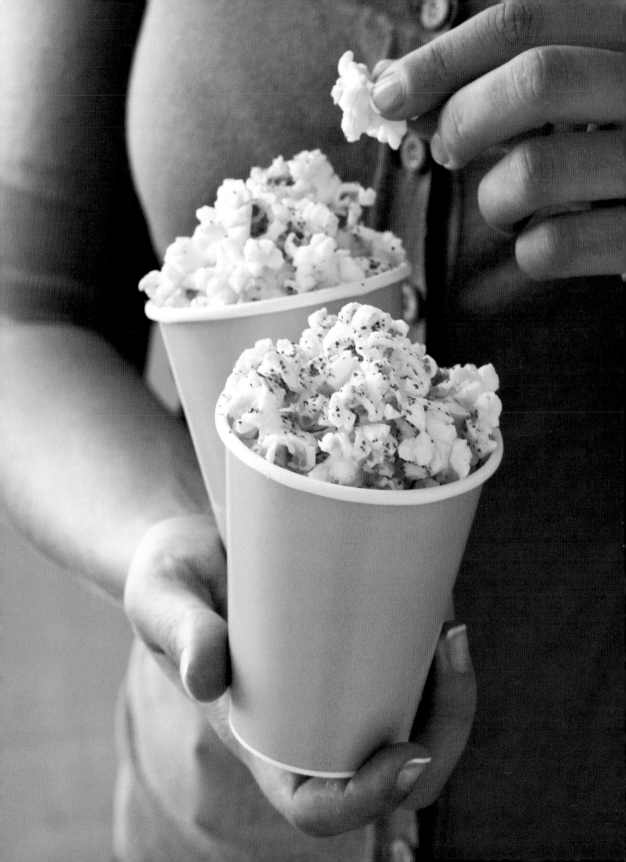

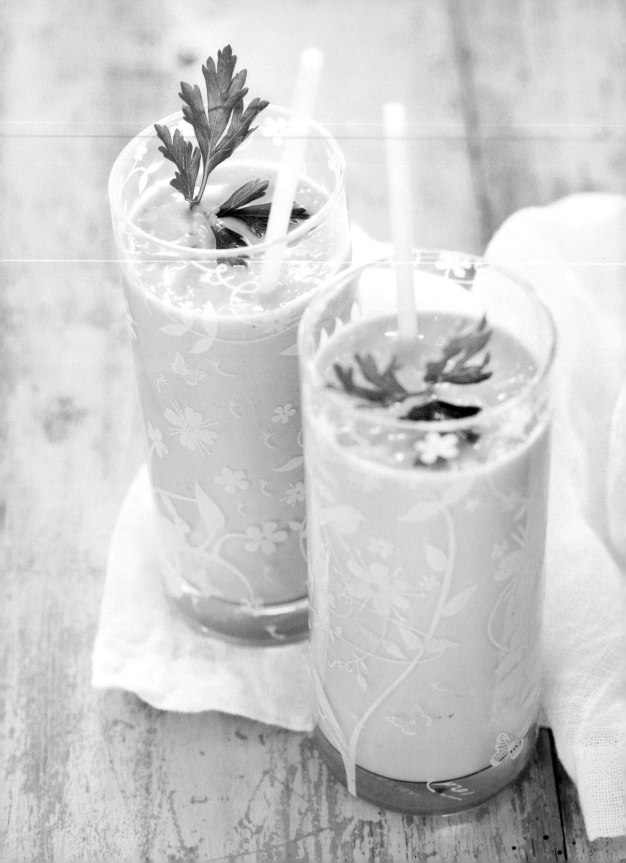

Go Green Smoothie

4 servings
(1 cup / 240 ml per serving)

PREP: 10 minutes

TOTAL: 10 minutes

When I need an instant pick-me-up, I make this smoothie – it's like drinking health in a glass. Don't be afraid of the color! It may be green but it doesn't taste that way – pineapple sweetens the blend while avocado gives it a decadent thickness.

Ingredients

1 bunch kale

1 bunch parsley

½ cup / 120 ml wheat grass

½ fresh pineapple, roughly chopped

1 piece ginger, about the size of your thumb

1 lime

½ avocado

1 cup / 240 ml unsweetened almond milk

¼ cup / 60 ml organic hemp protein powder with fiber ✱

Note: You will need a juicer or a blender for this recipe.

✱ You can find this product at health food stores, or online at www.livingharvest.com or www.manitobaharvest.com

Nutritional Value Per Serving:
Calories: 223 | Calories from Fat: 58 | Protein: 11 g | Carbs: 34 g | Total Fat: 7 g | Saturated Fat: 0.8 g | Trans Fat: 0 g | Fiber: 13 g | Sodium: 110 mg | Cholesterol: 0 mg | Sugar: 9 g

Juicer Method

1 Using a juicer, juice kale, parsley, wheat grass, pineapple, ginger and lime. Pour juice into a blender and add avocado, almond milk and hemp powder. Blend until combined. Pour into a glass and enjoy!

Blender Method

1 Using a blender, blend all ingredients until smooth. Blending (instead of juicing) will leave you with a thick, fibrous drink. Add more almond milk if you prefer a smoother beverage.

No-Bake Power Balls ✪

10 servings

PREP: 10 minutes

TOTAL: 10 minutes

I've never met anyone who didn't like a power ball. They take no time at all to make, they're easy to transport, they crush hunger cravings, and kids and adults alike adore their sweet and crunchy flavor. These balls are not part of your *Stripped* plan to lose that last 10, but don't worry — you'll love them even more while wearing your skinny jeans!

Ingredients

½ cup / 120 ml uncooked rolled oats

¼ cup / 60 ml pumpkin seeds

¼ cup / 60 ml dried unsweetened cranberries

¼ cup / 60 ml dried unsweetened currants

¼ cup / 60 ml organic hemp protein powder with fiber

¼ cup / 60 ml millet

2 Tbsp / 30 ml roasted golden whole flaxseed

½ cup / 120 ml natural nut butter

1 Tbsp / 15 ml unsulfured blackstrap molasses

½ tsp / 2.5 ml real vanilla

Nutritional Value Per Serving:

Calories: 188 | Calories from Fat: 79 | Protein: 8 g | Carbs: 19 g | Total Fat: 9 g | Saturated Fat: 1 g | Trans Fat: 0 g | Fiber: 5.7 g | Sodium: 4 mg | Cholesterol: 0 mg | Sugar: 6.8 g

Method

1   Combine all dry ingredients in a medium-sized bowl, mixing well. Stir in nut butter, molasses and vanilla. Using your hands, knead mixture until well combined.

2   Using an ice cream scooper, portion out 10 equal-sized balls and place in an airtight container. Store in refrigerator or freezer. No need to thaw before eating.

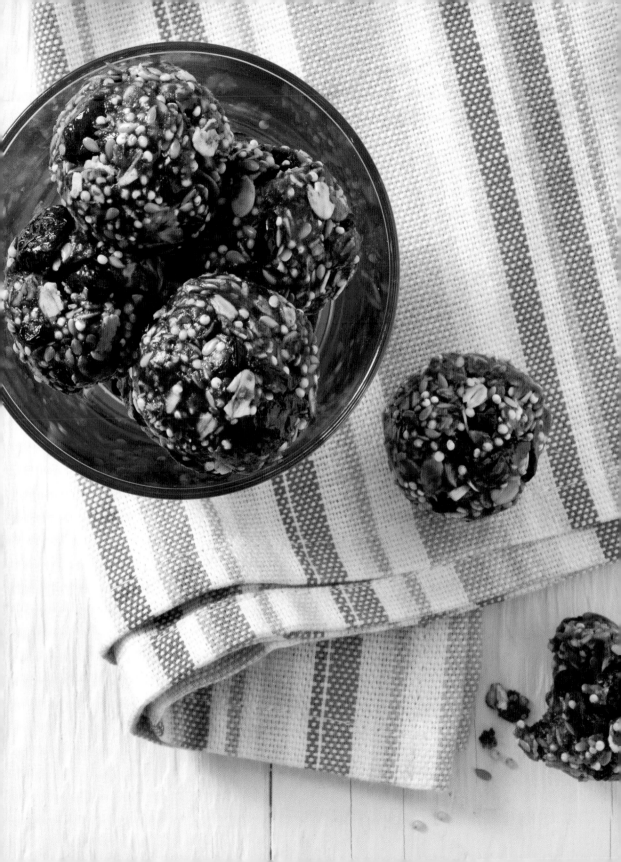

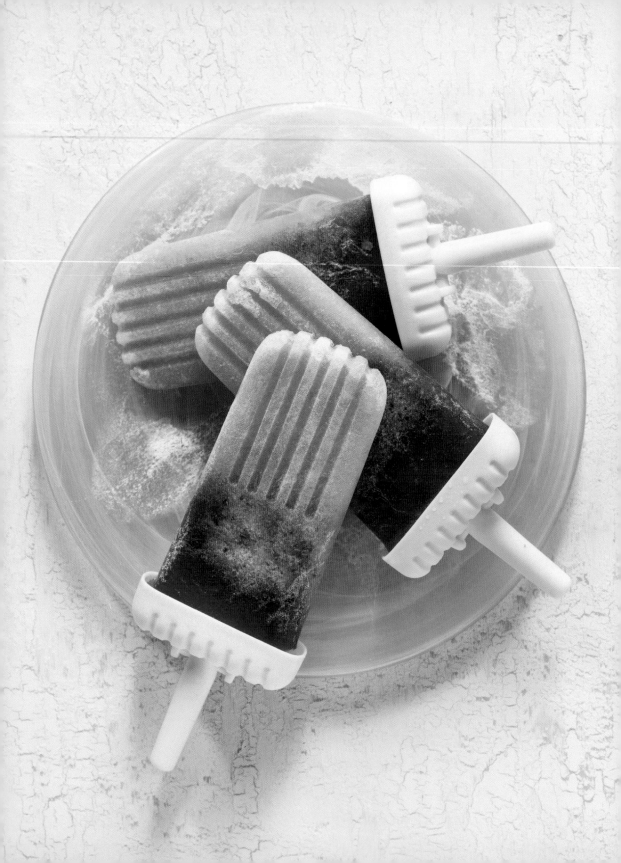

Keep it Cool Cucumber Melon Ice Pops

It's so easy (and so much healthier!) to make your own ice pops. These simple suckers feel like a decadent treat, but don't consist of anything other than fruits and vegetables! What a good way to sneak more nutrients into your – and your family's – diet.

Ingredients

1 cup / 240 ml English chopped cucumber

1 cup / 240 ml chopped Tuscan-style ripe cantaloupe

1 cup / 240 ml chopped ripe seedless watermelon

Note: You will need ice pop molds for this recipe.

Nutritional Value Per Serving:

Calories: 19 | Calories from Fat: 1 | Protein: 0.5 g | Carbs: 4.7 g | Total Fat: 0 g | Saturated Fat: 0 g | Trans Fat: 0 g | Fiber: 0.5 g | Sodium: 5 mg | Cholesterol: 0 mg | Sugar: 4 g

Method

1 In a food processor, process cucumber until blended. Pour into a small bowl and set aside. Rinse out the food processor and repeat with cantaloupe and watermelon, keeping each separate.

2 Place ice pop molds in their tray to stay upright. Spoon in blended cantaloupe, then cucumber and then watermelon to create three layers filling up each ice pop mold. Alternate the order to create different color combinations, if desired.

3 Put molds in freezer for at least three hours or until completely frozen. To serve, hold ice pop molds sideways under warm running water until they loosen.

Light and Lean Leek and Potato Soup

4 servings
(1¾ cups / 420 ml per serving)

PREP: 10 minutes

TOTAL: 35 minutes

This classic soup is a favorite of many – it's tasty, the texture is very pleasant and as a bonus it's also economical. Delicious served hot or cold, I like to make a big pot on Sunday and save the leftovers for weekday lunches.

Ingredients

1 tsp / 5 ml olive oil

2 leeks, white and light green parts only, cleaned and thinly sliced

3 small zucchini, thinly sliced

2 cloves garlic, chopped

1 Tbsp / 15 ml chopped fresh thyme

½ Tbsp / 7.5 ml sea salt

½ tsp / 2.5 ml freshly ground black pepper

1 russet potato, peeled and cut into 1-inch chunks

4 cups / 960 ml reduced-sodium chicken or vegetable broth

Juice of 1 lemon (2 to 3 Tbsp / 30 to 45 ml)

Snipped fresh chives, to garnish

Nutritional Value Per Serving:

Calories: 145 | Calories from Fat: 13 | Protein: 4 g | Carbs: 31 g | Total Fat: 1.5 g | Saturated Fat: 0 g | Trans Fat: 0 g | Fiber: 4 g | Sodium: 930 mg | Cholesterol: 0 mg | Sugar: 6 g

Method

1 Heat olive oil in a large soup pot over medium-high heat. Add leeks and cook until soft, about three minutes. Add zucchini, garlic, thyme, salt and pepper, and cook two minutes.

2 Add potato and stock. Bring to a boil, cover and reduce heat to simmer until vegetables are tender, 20 minutes.

3 Using an immersion blender, food processor or stand blender, blend soup until very smooth, working in batches if necessary. Add lemon juice, taste and make any final adjustments to seasoning with salt and pepper.

4 Ladle into bowls and top with fresh chives.

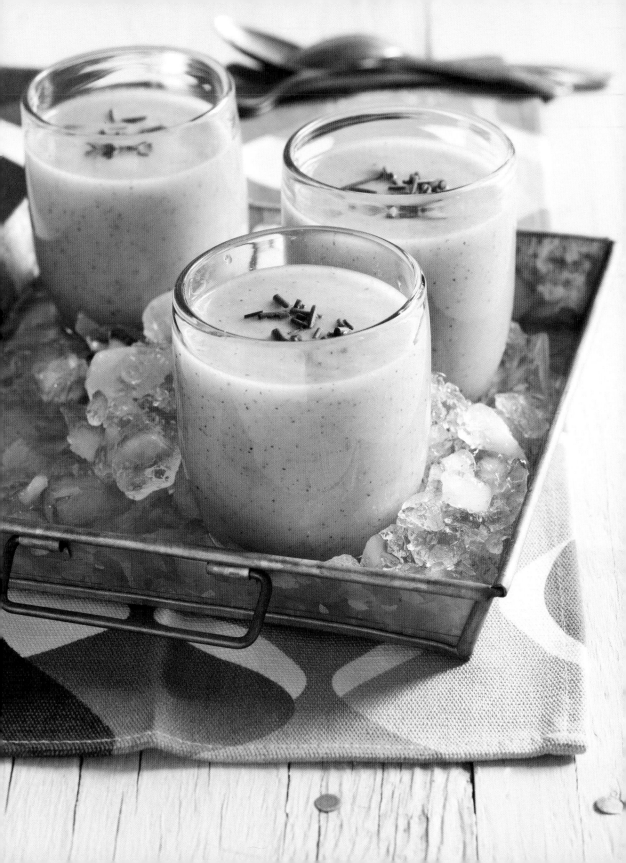

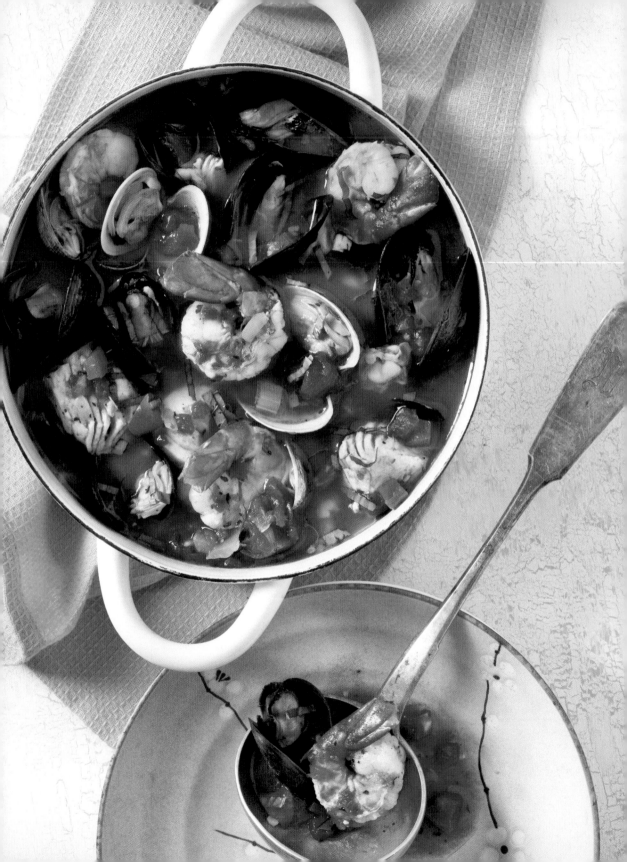

Easy Emerald City Bouillabaisse

4 servings
(2 ½ cups / 600 ml per serving)

PREP: 10 minutes

TOTAL: 40 minutes

Known for its simplicity, bouillabaisse is a classic French seafood and fish stew. The fresher your seafood, the better your bouillabaisse will be.

Ingredients

1 tsp / 5 ml olive oil

1 yellow onion, finely chopped

3 stalks celery, finely chopped

1 red pepper, seeded and finely chopped

½ Tbsp / 7.5 ml sea salt

½ tsp / 2.5 ml freshly ground black pepper

3 cloves garlic, finely chopped

½ tsp / 2.5 ml dried Italian herbs

1 tsp / 5 ml fennel seeds

½ tsp / 2.5 ml ground cumin

¼ tsp / 1.25 ml cayenne pepper

1 bay leaf

4 cups / 960 ml reduced-sodium chicken broth

1 x 14½-oz can no-salt-added diced tomatoes

6 large wild-caught prawns, peeled and deveined

12 manila clams, scrubbed (about ½ lb / 227 g)

12 mussels, debearded (about ½ lb / 227 g)

1 lb / 454 g halibut, cod or similar fish, cut into 2-inch chunks

Juice of 1 lemon (2 to 3 Tbsp / 30 to 45 ml)

¼ cup / 60 ml thinly sliced fresh basil

Nutritional Value Per Serving:

Calories: 375 | Calories from Fat: 67 | Protein: 51 g | Carbs: 26 g | Total Fat: 5 g | Saturated Fat: 0.3 g | Trans Fat: 0 g | Fiber: 6 g | Sodium: 1546 mg | Cholesterol: 110 mg | Sugar: 4 g

Method

1　Heat olive oil in a large pot over medium heat. Add onion, celery, red pepper, salt and pepper and cook until vegetables soften, about five minutes. Stir in garlic, Italian herbs, fennel seed, cumin, cayenne and bay leaf, and cook for two more minutes.

2　Add broth and tomatoes. Bring to a boil, cover and reduce heat to simmer for 20 minutes.

3　Uncover and increase heat so liquid is briskly simmering, but not boiling. Add seafood, cover, and cook for three to four minutes until halibut is opaque, shrimp are slightly curled, and clams and mussels are open. Discard any mussels or clams that do not open.

4　Stir in lemon juice and serve in large, shallow bowls topped with fresh basil.

Tasty Naked Wonton Soup

4 servings

PREP: 10 minutes

TOTAL: 35 minutes

The word "wonton" literally means "eating clouds" in Cantonese. In wonton soup, cooked wontons are meant to resemble fluffy, soft pillows floating in broth – just like clouds. This soup is typically made with wonton skins, a mix of flour, water and occasionally egg, but in this lighter version, the wontons are bursting with flavor and floating free.

Ingredients

8 cups / 1920 ml low-sodium chicken broth

1 Tbsp / 15 ml thinly sliced ginger (heaping)

2 cloves garlic, thinly sliced

1 whole star anise

1 bunch green onions, chopped, dark green parts divided from the white and light green parts

1 tsp / 5 ml sea salt, divided

1 lb / 454 g extra lean ground chicken

1 Tbsp / 15 ml reduced-sodium tamari

1 tsp / 5 ml sesame oil

¼ tsp / 1.25 ml Chinese five spice powder

¼ tsp / 1.25 ml freshly ground black pepper

4 baby bok choy, cut in half lengthwise

Chili sauce, to garnish (optional)

Nutritional Value Per Serving (2 cups / 480 ml broth, 6 naked wontons, 1 baby bok choy):

Calories: 233 | Calories from Fat: 79 | Protein: 28.5 g | Carbs: 11 g | Total Fat: 9 g | Saturated Fat: 3 g | Trans Fat: 0 g | Fiber: 3 g | Sodium: 901 mg | Cholesterol: 99 mg | Sugar: 3 g

Method

1 In a large saucepot, combine chicken broth, ginger, garlic, star aniseed, and white and light green parts of green onions over high heat until boiling. Reduce heat to simmer until flavors combine, about 20 minutes. Strain broth into a large bowl; pour broth back into saucepot and return to stove over low heat. Season with half a teaspoon salt.

2 In the meantime, combine chicken, tamari, sesame oil, Chinese five spice, remaining half-teaspoon salt, pepper and half of dark green part of green onions. Mix well.

3 Increase temperature under strained broth to bring to a brisk simmer. Spoon out golf-ball-sized portions of ground chicken and add to simmering broth to cook through, about 5 minutes. Lay baby bok choy on top of naked wontons cut side down, cover; steam for one minute.

4 Split soup evenly between four large bowls. Top with remaining dark green onions and chili sauce, if desired.

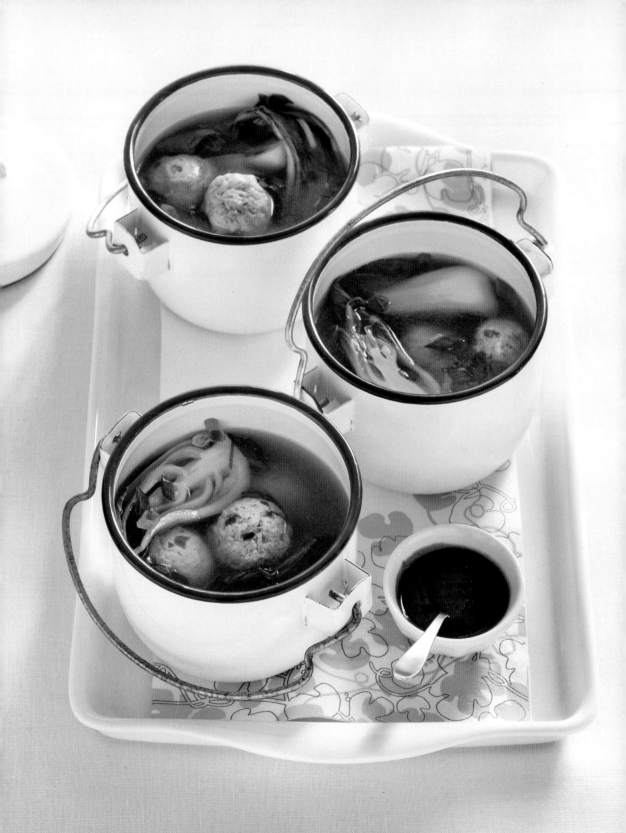

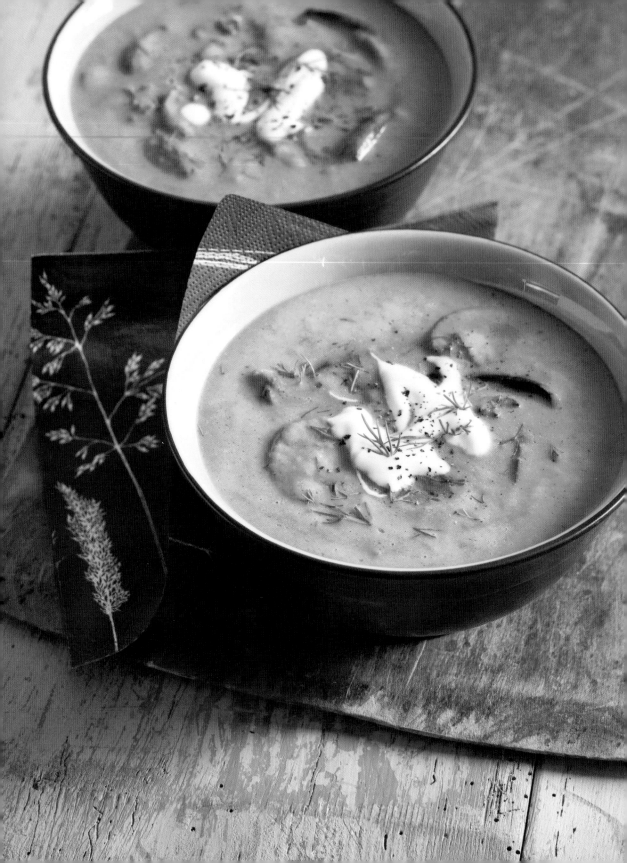

Makes Me 'Hungary' Hungarian Mushroom Soup

This soup may deceive you. It's hearty and meaty ... without actually containing any meat! This mushroom soup is warm, comforting and packed with nutrition. Perfect for an easy dinner on a chilly autumn evening.

Ingredients

1 tsp / 5 ml olive oil

1 onion, finely chopped

2 carrots, finely chopped

2 stalks celery, finely chopped

2 cloves garlic, finely chopped

1 tsp / 5 ml kosher salt

½ tsp / 2.5 ml freshly ground black pepper

1 Tbsp / 15 ml paprika

1 Tbsp / 15 ml whole wheat flour

6 cups / 1440 ml reduced-sodium mushroom or vegetable broth

2 tsp / 10 ml chopped fresh thyme

1 bay leaf

¼ cup / 60 ml unsweetened almond milk

½ lb / 227 g crimini mushrooms, sliced (about 4 cups / 960 ml)

2 portobello mushrooms, stems and gills removed, sliced into 2-inch pieces

1 tsp / 5 ml reduced-sodium tamari

2 Tbsp / 30 ml finely chopped fresh dill

Juice of ½ lemon (1 to 2 Tbsp / 15 to 30 ml)

Yogurt Cheese to garnish (optional, see page 301 for recipe)

Nutritional Value Per Serving:

Calories: 109 | Calories from Fat: 16 | Protein: 5 g | Carbs: 20 g | Total Fat: 1.7 g | Saturated Fat: 0 g | Trans Fat: 0 g | Fiber: 6 g | Sodium: 612 mg | Cholesterol: 0 mg | Sugar: 8.5 g

Method

1 Heat olive oil in a large pot over medium-high heat. Add onion, carrots, celery, garlic, salt and pepper, and cook until soft, stirring occasionally, five minutes.

2 Add paprika and flour, and stir to coat the vegetables. Add broth, thyme and bay leaf. Bring to a boil, reduce heat and simmer uncovered for 20 minutes.

3 Remove bay leaf and add almond milk. Blend soup with an immersion blender or stand blender, working in batches if necessary.

4 Return soup to pot and place on stove over medium-high heat. Stir in mushrooms, cover and reduce heat to simmer, 10 minutes.

5 Stir in tamari, dill and lemon juice. Taste and make any final adjustments to seasoning.

6 To serve, ladle into bowls, and if desired, top with fresh dill and Yogurt Cheese (omit if you are following the *Stripped* plan).

Lots o' Peppers Seafood and Black Bean Chili

6 servings
(1¾ cups / 420 ml per serving)

PREP: 15 minutes

TOTAL: 50 minutes

Traditional chili recipes are made with ground beef and tons of tomatoes. This colorful seafood chili is a much lighter – and much more interesting – variation. Try it as is, or serve over brown rice or spinach for a more filling fiesta.

Ingredients

1 tsp / 5 ml olive oil

1 onion, finely chopped

1 green pepper, seeded and chopped

1 red pepper, seeded and chopped

1 poblano pepper, seeded and chopped

2 cloves garlic, chopped

½ Tbsp / 7.5 ml sea salt

½ tsp / 2.5 ml freshly ground black pepper

2 chipotle peppers in adobo sauce, finely chopped

1 tsp / 5 ml ground cumin

½ tsp / 2.5 ml ground coriander

1 tsp / 5 ml chili powder

1 Tbsp / 15 ml fresh oregano, or 1 tsp / 5 ml dried

1 bay leaf

2 x 15-oz cans black beans, drained and rinsed

3 cups / 720 ml reduced-sodium chicken broth

1 x 28-oz can no-salt-added diced tomatoes

1 lb / 454 g mild fish (rock fish, cod or halibut), cut into 1-inch chunks

½ lb / 227 g cooked bay shrimp

Yogurt Cheese to garnish (optional, see page 301 for recipe)

Fresh cilantro, to garnish

1 lime, cut into wedges

Nutritional Value Per Serving:

Calories: 313 | Calories from Fat: 45 | Protein: 32 g | Carbs: 34 g | Total Fat: 5 g | Saturated Fat: 0.5 g | Trans Fat: 0 g | Fiber: 11 g | Sodium: 690 mg | Cholesterol: 98 mg | Sugar: 7 g

Method

1   Heat oil in a large soup pot over medium-high heat. Add onion, green, red and poblano peppers, garlic, salt and pepper, and cook until soft, 10 minutes. Add chipotle peppers with sauce, cumin, coriander, chili powder, oregano, bay leaf, beans, broth and tomatoes. Cover and simmer, 20 minutes.

2   Uncover, remove bay leaf and discard. Increase heat so liquid is briskly simmering. Add fish and gently submerge it into chili using a spoon. Allow fish to cook for three to four minutes until opaque. Taste chili and season with salt and pepper, to taste.

3   Ladle chili into bowls, top with bay shrimp, Yogurt Cheese (skip if you are following the *Stripped* plan) and cilantro. Serve with lime wedges to squeeze overtop.

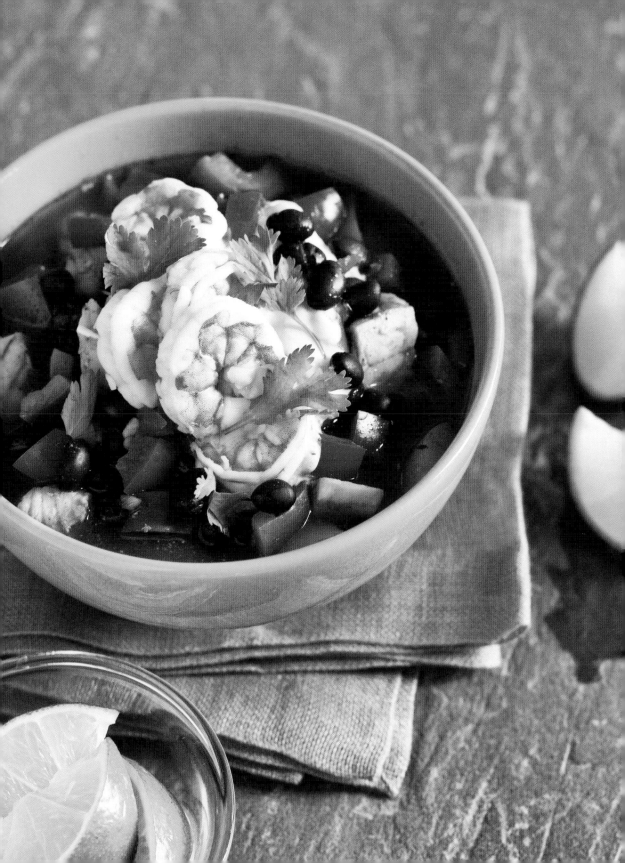

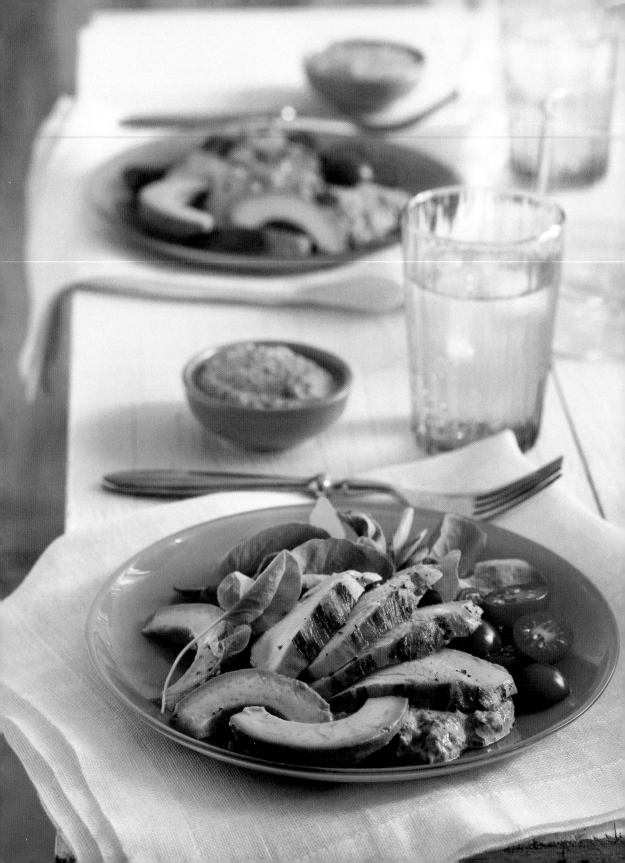

Country Club Watercress and Grilled Chicken Salad with Putting Green Dressing

SALAD:
2 servings

PREP: 15 minutes

TOTAL: 21 to 25 minutes

DRESSING:
¾ cup / 180 ml

PREP: 5 minutes

TOTAL: 5 minutes

After a grueling 18 holes of golf, you need to refuel. Enter this classy Country Club Salad. It's a composed salad, which means that the ingredients are arranged in little piles on the plate, rather than being tossed together. The result is nothing short of elegance!

Ingredients

SALAD:
Eat-Clean Cooking Spray
    (see page 214 for recipe)
8 oz / 227 g chicken breasts
Sea salt and freshly ground
    black pepper, to taste
1 bunch (about 1½ cups / 360 ml)
    watercress
4 to 6 Tbsp / 60 to 90 ml dressing
    (recipe to the right)
½ cup / 120 ml halved cherry or
    grape tomatoes
½ avocado, thinly sliced

DRESSING✻ :
1 tsp / 5 ml chopped shallots
½ tsp / 1.25 ml chopped garlic
¼ cup / 60 ml chopped fresh chives
¼ cup / 60 ml chopped fresh basil
¼ cup / 60 ml chopped fresh parsley
½ tsp / 2.5 ml anchovy paste
½ cup / 120 ml Yogurt Cheese
    (see page 301 for recipe)
½ tsp / 120 ml sea salt
⅛ tsp / pinch freshly ground
    black pepper
Juice of ½ fresh lemon
    (1 to 2 Tbsp / 15 to 30 ml)

✻ Unused dressing will last up to one week in the refrigerator.

Note: If you are following the *Stripped* plan, skip the dressing and use a spritz of balsamic vinegar and lemon juice.

Nutritional Value for ¹/₂ recipe (with 3 Tbsp / 45 ml dressing):

Calories: 226 | Calories from Fat: 76 | Protein: 27 g | Carbs: 6.6 g | Total Fat: 7 g | Saturated Fat: 1 g | Trans Fat: 0 g | Fiber: 3.75 g | Sodium: 236 mg | Cholesterol: 64 mg | Sugar: 1.7 g

Method

SALAD:

1   Heat a grill or grill pan to medium-high heat and coat with Eat-Clean Cooking Spray. Season both sides of chicken with salt and pepper and place on grill. Cook three to five minutes on each side until done. Remove to a cutting board to rest for three minutes. Thinly slice on the diagonal.

2   Divide watercress between two large plates. Drizzle 2 to 3 Tbsp / 30 to 45 ml dressing over watercress stems on each plate, and fan out sliced chicken overtop. On one side of each plate, pile cherry tomatoes and on other side, fan out avocado slices.

DRESSING (OPTIONAL):

1   Add dressing ingredients, except for lemon juice, to a food processor and pulse to combine. While processor is running, stream in lemon juice until thick and blended (you may not need all lemon juice). Scrape into a bowl and set aside.

Ladies' Lunch Quick Shrimp Ceviche Stuffed Avocados

4 servings
(1 cup / 240 ml ceviche +
½ avocado per serving)

PREP: 25 minutes

TOTAL: 25 minutes

Ceviche, a seafood dish that is popular in South America, is typically made with raw fish marinated in citrus juices. Here I've used cooked shrimp and paired it with avocado. Ceviche also complements the flavors of sweet potatoes, lettuce and corn, so try them all before choosing a favorite.

Ingredients

1 lb / 454 g jumbo cooked shrimp, peeled and deveined

½ red pepper, seeded and finely chopped

¼ cup / 60 ml finely chopped red onion

¼ cup / 60 ml finely chopped green onion

½ jalapeno pepper, seeded and finely chopped

1 tomato, finely chopped

2 Tbsp / 30 ml chopped cilantro

Juice of ½ orange (about ⅛ cup / 30 ml)

Juice of 2 limes (4 to 6 Tbsp / 60 to 90 ml)

½ tsp / 2.5 ml sea salt

¼ tsp / 1.25 ml freshly ground black pepper

2 avocados

Nutritional Value Per Serving:

Calories: 301 | Calories from Fat: 136 | Protein: 26 g | Carbs: 15 g | Total Fat: 16 g | Saturated Fat: 2.5 g | Trans Fat: 0 g | Fiber: 8 g | Sodium: 463 mg | Cholesterol: 220 mg | Sugar: 4 g

Method

1 Remove shrimp tails and discard. Cut each shrimp into three or four pieces. In a bowl, combine shrimp with all other ingredients except avocados. Refrigerate for 15 minutes to allow flavors to combine.

2 Cut avocados in half and remove pits. Using a large spoon, scoop avocados out of their skins. Spoon ceviche into center of each avocado half, allowing it to overflow. Serve immediately.

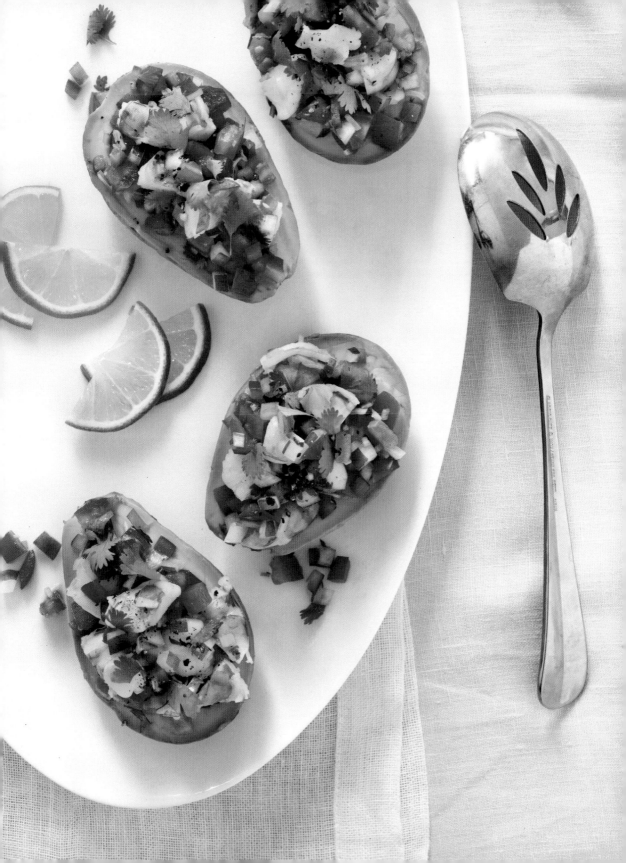

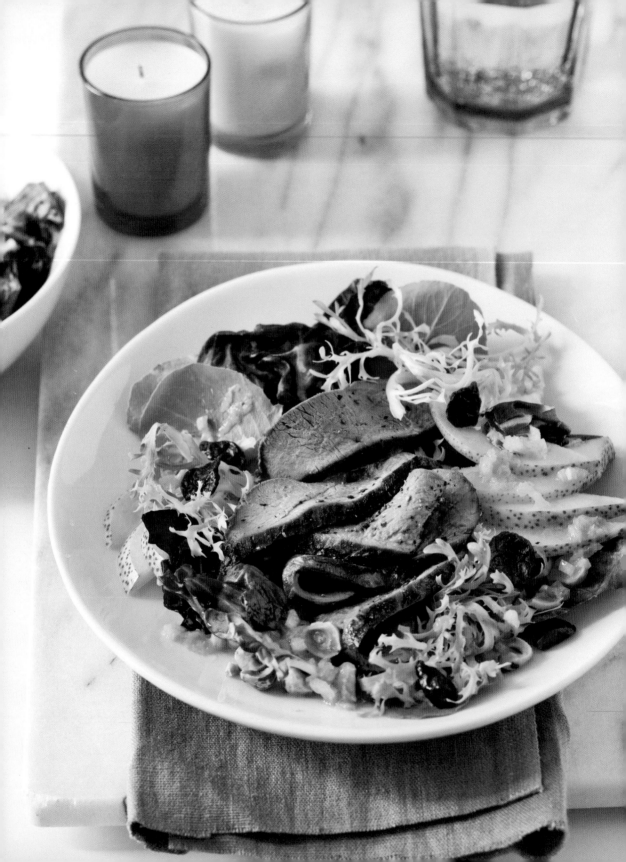

Ode to Oregon Grilled Duck and Bitter Greens Salad with Pears, Dried Cherries and Hazelnuts

4 servings

PREP: 20 minutes

TOTAL: 33 minutes

This salad tastes so gourmet, I wouldn't be surprised to find it on the menu in an upscale, pricey restaurant. With this recipe, you can make it – and enjoy it – at home for a fraction of the cost.

Nutritional Value Per Serving:

Calories: 417 | Calories from Fat: 197 | Protein: 21 g | Carbs: 32 g | Total Fat: 23 g | Saturated Fat: 3 g | Trans Fat: 0 g | Fiber: 6.5 g | Sodium: 489 mg | Cholesterol: 64 mg | Sugar: 20 g

Ingredients

SALAD:

½ cup / 120 ml roasted hazelnuts

2 x 8 oz boneless duck breasts, skin removed

Sea salt and freshly ground black pepper

1 head radicchio, core removed and cut into large bite-sized pieces

4 cups / 960 ml escarole, torn into large bite-sized pieces

4 cups / 960 ml frisée, torn into large bite-sized pieces

½ cup / 120 ml dried unsweetened pitted cherries (optional)

1 pear, cored, halved and thinly sliced

Eat-Clean Cooking Spray (see page 214 for recipe)

VINAIGRETTE:

2 Tbsp / 30 ml red wine vinegar

¼ large orange, zested and juiced

½ tsp / 2.5 ml Dijon mustard

1 tsp / 5 ml finey chopped shallots

½ tsp / 2.5 ml sea salt

¼ tsp / 1.25 ml freshly ground black pepper

2 Tbsp / 30 ml hazelnut or walnut oil

Method

SALAD:

1 Preheat oven to 350°F / 175°C. Place hazelnuts on a baking sheet and roast in oven, five minutes. Remove, let cool a few minutes, then roughly chop.

2 Heat a grill or grill pan to medium-high heat and spray with Eat-Clean Cooking Spray. Season both sides of duck with salt and pepper. Lay duck presentation side down (side where skin was removed) on grill. Cook duck two to three minutes then rotate 45 degrees (for example, from 12 to two on a clock) and cook for an additional two to three minutes to create crosshatch marks and to prevent burning. Flip duck and repeat, cooking to desired doneness, eight minutes total cooking time for medium rare (this is safe with duck) or up to 12 minutes total cooking time for medium to medium well.

3 Combine radicchio, escarole, frisée and cherries (skip the cherries if you are following the *Stripped* plan) in a large bowl. Pour dressing (method below) over top and toss to combine.

4 To serve, divide salad equally among four plates. Thinly slice duck on the bias and fan out on one side of each salad. Divide pear slices equally among plates and fan out opposite duck.

VINAIGRETTE:

1 Whisk together all vinaigrette ingredients, except oil. While whisking, drizzle in oil.

Sweetheart Shrimp and Watermelon Salad

The first time someone told me about pairing shrimp and water-melon in the same dish, I was skeptical, but this is a match made in Eat-Clean heaven! The sweetness of the melon balances the slight salty flavor of the shrimp. Serve it up to your sweetheart tonight!

Ingredients

4 cups / 960 ml ripe seedless watermelon, rind removed and cut into bite-sized pieces

2 Tbsp / 30 ml white balsamic vinegar

1 tsp / 5 ml Dijon mustard

½ tsp / 2.5 ml salt, divided

½ tsp / 2.5 ml freshly ground black pepper, divided

1 Tbsp / 15 ml watermelon juice (see directions below)

1 Tbsp / 15 ml extra virgin olive oil

Eat-Clean Cooking Spray (see page 214 for recipe)

1 lb / 454 g wild jumbo shrimp, shelled and deveined

2 cloves of garlic, minced

4 cups / 960 ml packed baby spinach

4 cups / 960 ml frisée, torn into large bite-sized pieces

¼ red onion, thinly sliced

1 cup / 240 ml grape or cherry tomatoes

Nutritional Value Per Serving:

Calories: 220 | Calories from Fat: 46 | Protein: 27 g | Carbs: 18 g | Total Fat: 3.5 g | Saturated Fat: 0.5 g | Trans Fat: 0 g | Fiber: 3 g | Sodium: 558 mg | Cholesterol: 220 mg | Sugar: 13 g

Method

1 Place cut watermelon in a bowl and set aside. In a small bowl, add vinegar, Dijon mustard, honey, ¼ tsp / 1.25 ml salt and ¼ tsp / 1.25 ml black pepper. Strain 1 Tbsp / 15 ml watermelon juice that has collected in bottom of watermelon bowl into small bowl containing vinaigrette ingredients. Whisk to combine and while whisking, drizzle in olive oil and set aside.

2 Heat a large nonstick skillet over medium heat and coat with Eat-Clean Cooking Spray. Add shrimp, remaining ¼ tsp / 1.25 ml salt and ¼ tsp / 1.25 ml black pepper. Sauté for three minutes and flip over. Spray with more Eat-Clean Cooking Spray, add garlic and sauté two more minutes or until cooked through.

3 In a large bowl, combine spinach, frisée and red onion. Drizzle half of vinaigrette over greens and toss to combine. Divide evenly among four plates and top with cherry tomatoes, watermelon and shrimp. Drizzle remaining dressing over top of each salad.

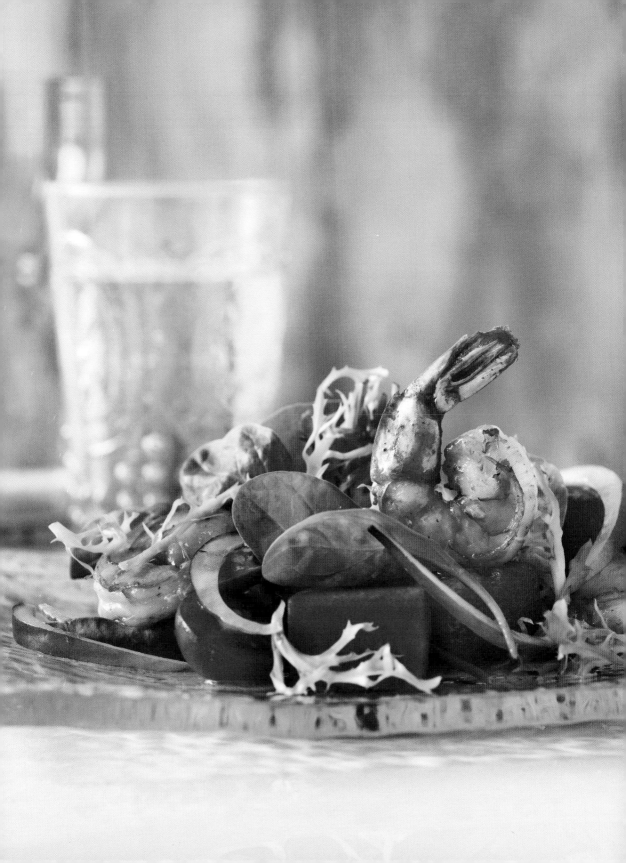

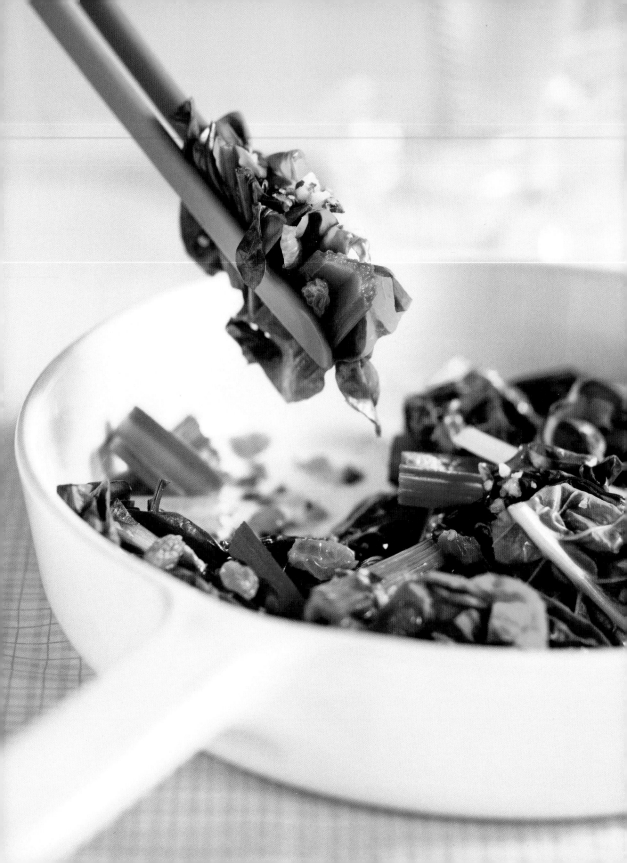

Sassy Southern Greens

High in vitamins and minerals, greens have been a staple food in the American South for a long time. American slaves would take the discarded tops of turnips and beets and simmer them in a pot, occasionally with a hog's foot added for flavor! Today these greens are popular both at home and in fancy restaurants.

Ingredients

1 tsp / 5 ml olive oil

⅛ tsp / pinch crushed red pepper flakes

2 cloves garlic, chopped

12 cups / 2880 ml chopped greens (such as collard, kale, mustard or beet)

2 Tbsp / 30 ml golden raisins (optional)

¼ tsp / 1.25 ml sea salt

⅛ tsp / pinch freshly ground black pepper

¼ cup / 60 ml low-sodium vegetable broth, or water

Nutritional Value Per Serving:

Calories: 101 | Calories from Fat: 17 | Protein: 5 g | Carbs: 19.5 g | Total Fat: 2 g | Saturated Fat: 0 g | Trans Fat: 0 g | Fiber: 4 g | Sodium: 161 mg | Cholesterol: 0 mg | Sugar: 4.5 g

Method

1 Heat olive oil in a very large nonstick skillet over medium-high heat. Add crushed red pepper flakes and garlic, and cook for 30 seconds until garlic becomes fragrant. Add greens, raisins (omit if following the *Stripped* plan), salt and pepper, and stir to combine. Stir in broth and cook until greens are wilted and tender crisp, about five minutes.

Fiesta Quinoa Pilaf

4 servings

PREP: 5 minutes

TOTAL: 30 minutes

In my mind quinoa is the perfect side dish (and occasional main course). It's commonly considered a grain, but it's actually a relative of leafy green vegetables such as spinach and Swiss chard. It adapts well to different flavors and exotic tastes from around the world – in this case, Spanish cuisine.

Ingredients

1 tsp / 5 ml olive oil

½ yellow onion, diced

½ yellow or orange pepper, seeded and diced

1 tsp / 5 ml sea salt

¼ tsp / 1.25 ml freshly ground black pepper

2 cloves garlic, minced

½ tsp / 2.5 ml ground cumin

½ tsp / 2.5 ml chili powder

⅛ tsp / pinch cayenne pepper

1 cup / 240 ml red quinoa, rinsed and drained

2 cups / 480 ml low-sodium vegetable or chicken broth

Juice of ½ lime (about 1 to 2 Tbsp / 15 to 30 ml)

¼ cup / 60 ml chopped scallions

¼ cup / 60 ml chopped fresh cilantro, plus more for garnish

Nutritional Value Per Serving:

Calories: 194 | Calories from Fat: 34 | Protein: 5.6 g | Carbs: 33 g | Total Fat: 3.7 g | Saturated Fat: 0 g | Trans Fat: 0 g | Fiber: 4 g | Sodium: 470 mg | Cholesterol: 0 mg | Sugar: 3 g

Method

1 Heat olive oil in a medium saucepan over medium-high heat. Add onion, pepper, salt and black pepper, and sauté until soft, three minutes. Stir in garlic, cumin, chili powder and cayenne, and cook for one more minute. Stir in quinoa and broth.

2 Cover, reduce heat and simmer for 15 to 20 minutes until all liquid is absorbed and quinoa is plumped up. Remove from heat, fluff with a fork, and let sit for five minutes, covered.

3 Stir in lime juice, scallions and cilantro; serve.

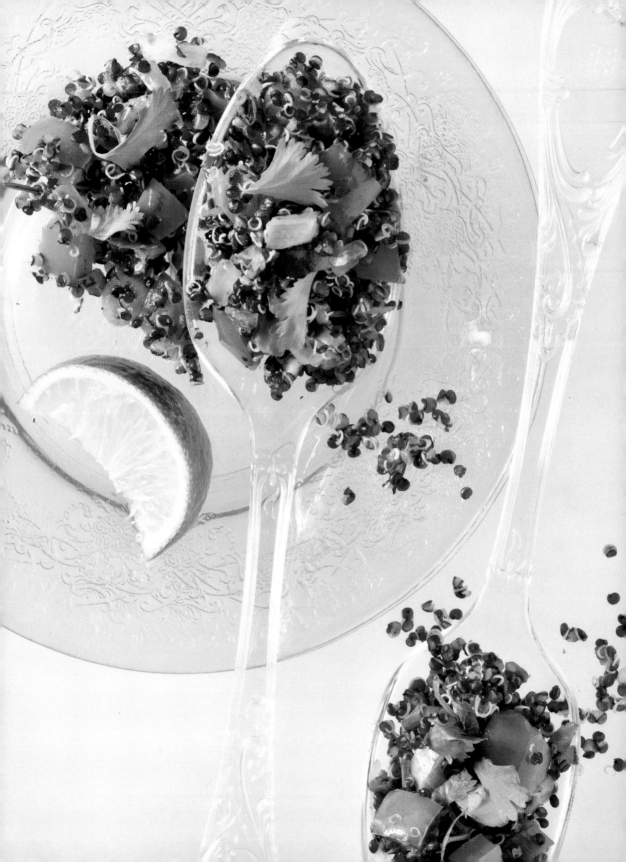

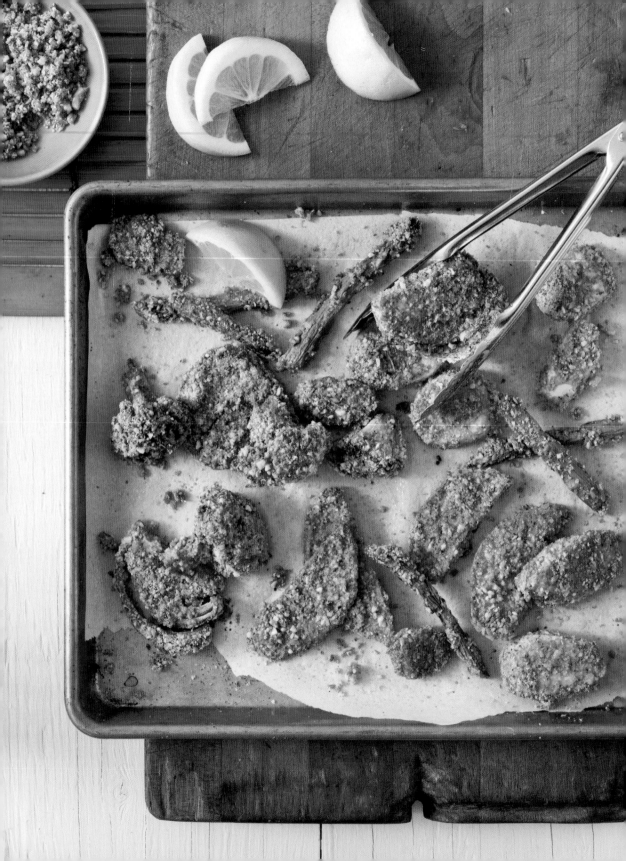

Eat Your Veggie Frites

4 servings

PREP: 15 minutes

TOTAL: 35 minutes

If you've only tried fries made from white potatoes, you're in for a treat. Kids and adults alike go crazy for these veggie frites. The best part? You can choose which veggies to roast based on what you've got on hand. It doesn't get any more convenient than that!

Ingredients

COATING:

1½ cups / 360 ml puffed whole grain kamut cereal

¼ cup / 60 ml oat bran

¼ cup / 60 ml raw cashews

1 Tbsp / 15 ml flaxseed

¾ tsp / 3.75 ml sea salt

1 tsp / 5 ml onion powder

¼ tsp / 1.25 ml garlic powder

¼ tsp / 1.25 ml celery seeds

¼ tsp / 1.25 sweet paprika

¼ tsp / 1.25 ml chili powder

¼ tsp / 1.25 ml freshly ground black pepper

EGG WASH:

2 egg whites

½ cup / 120 ml low-sodium vegetable broth or water

VEGGIES:

4 cups / 960 ml assorted vegetables, such as:

Asparagus, cut into 2-inch pieces

Sweet potatoes, peeled, cut in half lengthwise and sliced into ¼-inch pieces

Broccoli, cut into bite-sized pieces

Carrots, peeled and cut on the diagonal into ¼-inch coins

Parsnip, peeled and cut on the diagonal into ¼-inch coins

Sweet onions, peeled, quartered and sliced

Eat-Clean Cooking Spray (see page 214 for recipe)

Lemon wedges to garnish

Nutritional Value Per Serving ✳ :

Calories: 229 | Calories from Fat: 68 | Protein: 10 g | Carbs: 35 g | Total Fat: 7.5 g | Saturated Fat: 1 g | Trans Fat: 0 g | Fiber: 8 g | Sodium: 513 mg | Cholesterol: 0 mg | Sugar: 8 g

✳ NI based on ¼ cup / 60 ml sweet potatoes, ¼ cup / 60 ml broccoli, ¼ cup / 60 ml carrots and ¼ cup / 60 ml parsnips.

Method

1 Preheat oven to 400°F / 200°C. In a food processor, combine all coating ingredients and pulse until finely ground. Pour into a bowl and set aside.

2 In another bowl, whisk egg whites and vegetable stock until frothy and set aside.

3 Chop assorted veggies into bite-sized pieces similar in size.

4 Spray a baking sheet with Eat-Clean Cooking Spray. Working in batches, dip veggies into egg white mixture. Let excess drip off and place in coating mixture, flipping until completely covered. Shake off excess coating and place veggies on baking sheet. Spray lightly with Eat-Clean Cooking Spray.

5 Bake veggies for 20 minutes until golden brown. Serve with lemon wedges to squeeze overtop.

Vegetables à la Grecque

4 servings
(2 cups / 480 ml per serving)

PREP: 15 minutes

TOTAL: 265 minutes

With a name like "Vegetables à la Grecque," one would assume that this dish is native to Greece, but that is not the case. This recipe comes from France, where these vegetables are prepared in the Greek style. This means they are marinated in vinegar or lemon, olive oil and seasonings, then served cold after resting in the refrigerator.

Ingredients

2 cups / 480 ml distilled white vinegar

2 cups / 480 ml unfiltered apple cider vinegar

2 tsp / 10 ml coriander seeds

1 tsp / 5 ml whole black peppercorns

1 sprig fresh thyme

Few parsley stems

1 bay leaf

1 tsp / 5 ml sea salt

2 cups / 480 ml ice cubes

2 cloves garlic, slightly smashed

1 cup / 240 ml baby carrots

1 cup / 240 ml broccoli florets

1 cup / 240 ml cauliflower florets

1 cup / 240 ml white button mushrooms, quartered

½ English cucumber, cut into ½-inch thick coins

½ sweet onion, sliced

1 bulb fennel, sliced

Nutritional Value Per Serving:

Calories: 126 | Calories from Fat: 5 | Protein: 3.7 g | Carbs: 18 g | Total Fat: 0 g | Saturated Fat: 0 g | Trans Fat: 0 g | Fiber: 6 g | Sodium: 568 mg | Cholesterol: 0 mg | Sugar: 7 g

Method

1 In a small saucepan, combine vinegars, coriander seeds, black peppercorns, thyme, parsley stems, bay leaf and salt over medium high heat. Bring to boil, reduce heat and simmer gently for 10 minutes. Remove from heat, strain and add ice cubes.

2 Place garlic and vegetables in a large heatproof container and pour cooled vinegar mixture over top. Using a wooden spoon, gently press vegetables so they are submerged in liquid. If they can't all be submerged, stir vegetables after a couple of hours to make sure they all make contact with vinegar. Cover and refrigerate for at least four hours before serving. Vegetables will last up to five days in the refrigerator.

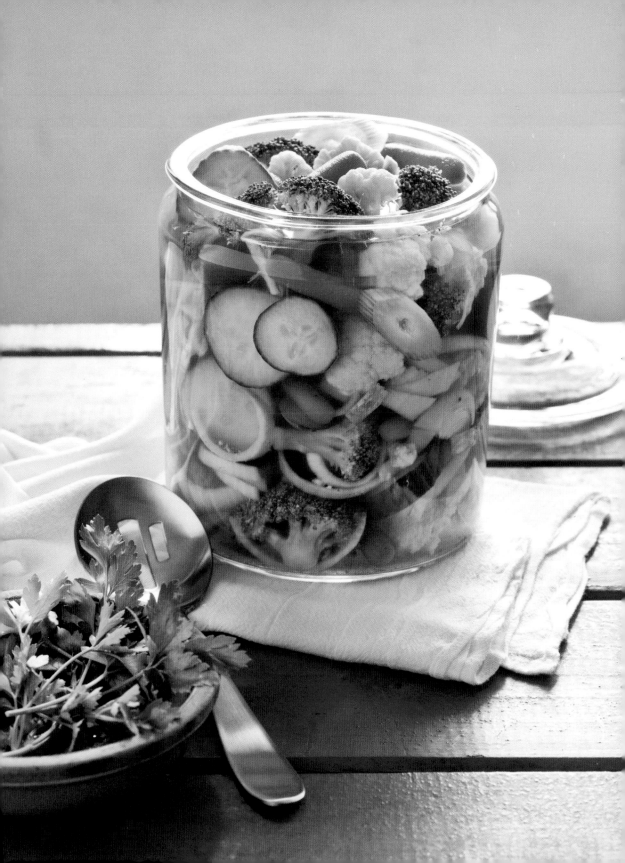

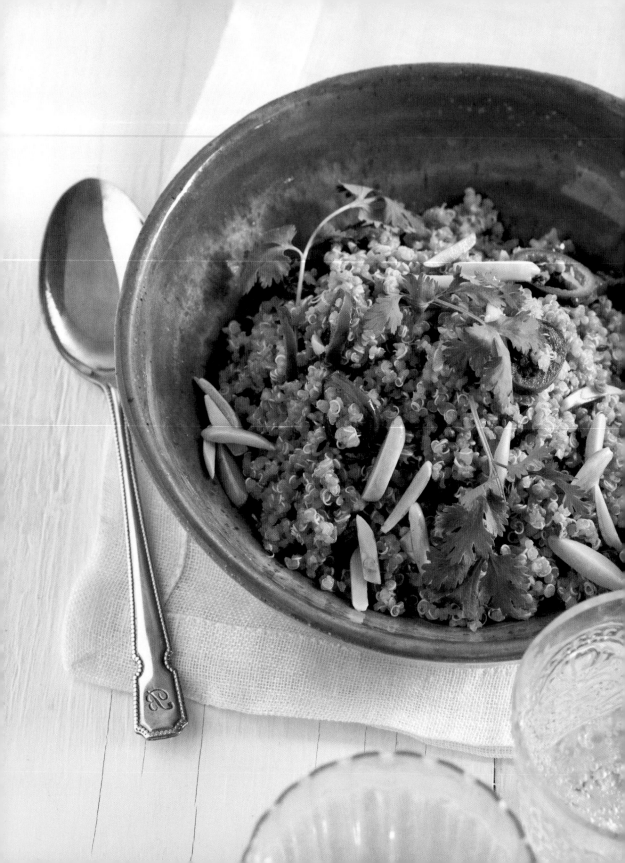

From India with Love Quinoa Pilaf

Whoever said healthy food had to be boring and bland never set foot into my kitchen. I love experimenting with spices and herbs from around the globe – it keeps mealtimes interesting and Clean. This recipe is inspired by Indian cuisine. For more info on herbs, turn to page 174.

Ingredients

1 tsp / 5 ml olive oil

1 tsp / 5 ml cumin seeds

¼ tsp / 1.25 ml coriander seeds

1 stick cinnamon

1 jalapeno, thinly sliced into circles

1 cup / 240 ml white quinoa, rinsed and drained

1 tsp / 5 ml ground turmeric

¼ tsp / 1.25 ml ground green cardamom

1 tsp / 5 ml sea salt

¼ tsp / 1.25 ml freshly ground black pepper

Juice of 1 lemon (about 2 to 3 Tbsp / 30 to 45 ml)

¼ cup / 60 ml chopped fresh cilantro

¼ cup / 60 ml toasted almond slivers

Nutritional Value Per Serving:

Calories: 215 | Calories from Fat: 62 | Protein: 6.5 g | Carbs: 31 g | Total Fat: 7 g | Saturated Fat: 0.6 g | Trans Fat: 0 g | Fiber: 4 g | Sodium: 396 mg | Cholesterol: 0 mg | Sugar: 1.5 g

Method

1   Heat olive oil in a large pot over medium-high heat. Add cumin seeds, coriander seeds, cinnamon stick and jalapeno, and sauté until fragrant, one minute. Add quinoa, turmeric and cardamom, and stir well with toasted spice mixture. Stir in two cups water, and salt and pepper. Bring to a boil, cover, reduce heat to low and simmer until all liquid is absorbed and quinoa is plumped, 10 to 15 minutes. Remove from heat, fluff, and let sit for five minutes, covered.

2   Stir in lemon juice, cilantro and almonds; serve.

Backyard BBQ Broccolini

4 servings

PREP: 5 minutes

TOTAL: 9 minutes

Broccolini is a green vegetable, similar to broccoli, but with long, thin stalks and small florets. Yellow flowers occasionally bloom on broccolini and the entire plant is edible. Try it sautéed, steamed, boiled and in stir-fries.

Ingredients

- 1 bunch broccolini, stem ends trimmed ½-inch
- ½ tsp / 2.5 ml olive oil
- ½ tsp / 2.5 ml onion powder
- ¼ tsp / 1.25 ml garlic powder
- ¼ tsp / 1.25 ml sea salt
- ⅛ tsp / pinch freshly ground black pepper

Nutritional Value Per Serving:

Calories: 20.6 | Calories from Fat: 5 | Protein: 1.4 g | Carbs: 1.8 g | Total Fat: 0.6 g | Saturated Fat: 0.1 g | Trans Fat: 0 g | Fiber: 1.4 g | Sodium: 131 mg | Cholesterol: 0 mg | Sugar: 0.2 g

Method

1 Heat a grill or grill pan to medium high. In a large bowl, toss together all ingredients until broccolini is thoroughly coated in seasonings.

2 Place broccolini on grill in a single layer and cook until slightly charred, about two minutes on each side.

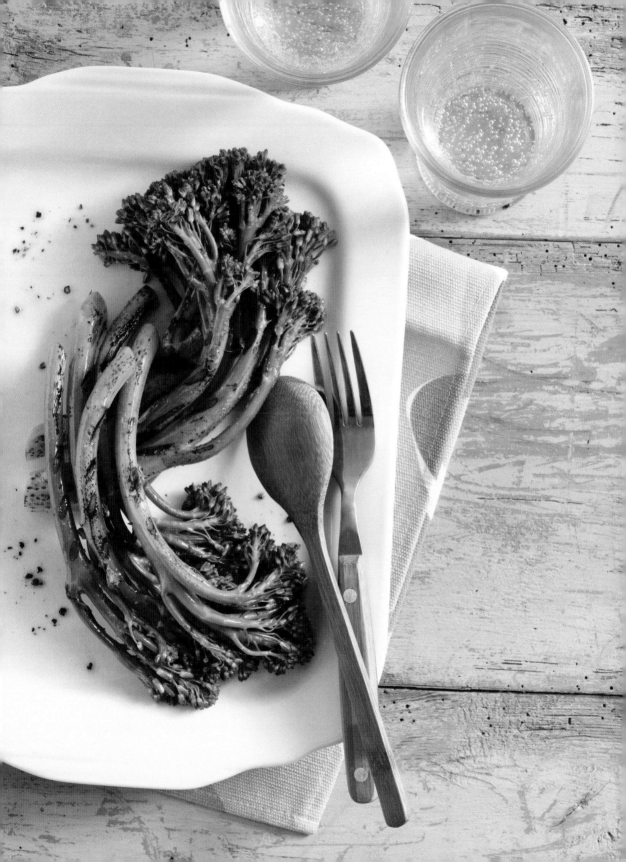

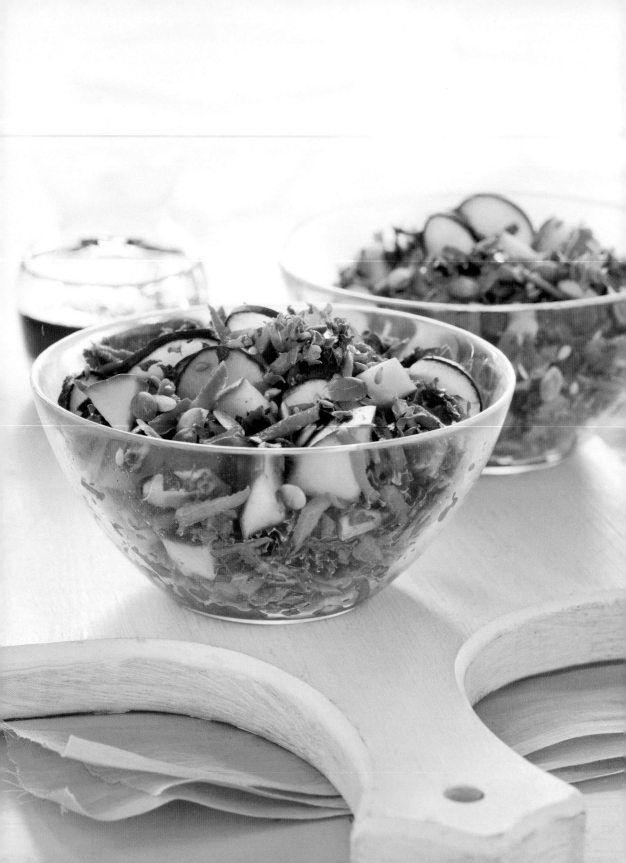

Your Body's Keen on Kale and Carrot Salad

If you haven't tried kale, you're missing out! It's an archaic type of cabbage that is very high in nutrients. It's known as a chewy green that tends to be slightly bitter in flavor, although this bitterness is lessened by using younger leaves, and washing and cooking the greens. Kale is a staple in my kitchen!

Ingredients

SALAD:
1 bunch kale leaves, stems removed (about 10 cups / 2400 ml packed)

2 carrots, peeled and grated

½ cup / 120 ml thinly sliced radishes

1 cup / 240 ml chopped English cucumber

2 Tbsp / 30 ml shelled raw pumpkin seeds

1 Tbsp / 15 ml golden roasted flaxseed

DRESSING:
2 Tbsp / 30 ml reduced-sodium tamari

2 Tbsp / 30 ml rice vinegar

2 tsp / 10 ml lime juice

2 tsp / 20 ml toasted sesame oil

1 clove garlic, minced

1 tsp / 5 ml grated ginger

¼ tsp / 1.25 ml ground cumin

⅛ tsp / pinch cayenne

¼ tsp / 1.25 ml sea salt

¼ tsp / 1.25 ml freshly ground black pepper

Nutritional Value Per Serving:

Calories: 172 | Calories from Fat: 58 | Protein: 9 g | Carbs: 23 g | Total Fat: 7 g | Saturated Fat: 1 g | Trans Fat: 0 g | Fiber: 6 g | Sodium: 548 mg | Cholesterol: 0 mg | Sugar: 2 g

Method

1 In a food processor, pulse kale leaves until coarsely chopped, working in batches if necessary. Place chopped kale into a large bowl and add carrots, radishes, cucumber and pumpkin seeds.

2 In a small bowl, whisk together all dressing ingredients. Pour over salad and toss to combine. Serve topped with flaxseed.

Basque-Style Green Beans

4 servings

PREP: 10 minutes

TOTAL: 20 minutes

Basque cuisine refers to the dishes created in the area of the border between France and Spain on the Atlantic coast. Food and cooking are very important in Basque culture, and this internationally popular cuisine typically contains sweet or hot peppers.

Ingredients

1 lb / 454 g green beans, ends trimmed

½ tsp / 2.5 ml olive oil

2 cloves garlic, finely chopped

½ red pepper, core removed and finely chopped

½ yellow pepper, core removed and finely chopped

¼ tsp / 1.25 ml kosher salt

⅛ tsp / pinch freshly ground black pepper

Nutritional Value Per Serving:

Calories: 54 | Calories from Fat: 5.8 |
Protein: 4.4 g | Carbs: 10.9 g |
Total Fat: 0.6 g | Saturated Fat: 0.1 g |
Trans Fat: 0 g | Fiber: 4.5 g |
Sodium: 80 mg | Cholesterol: 0 mg |
Sugar: 0.6 g

Method

1 Bring a large pot of water to boil over high heat. Add green beans and cook until bright green and tender-crisp, one to two minutes. Remove green beans from boiling water and submerge in a large bowl of ice water. Using tongs, remove from cold water and drain in a colander.

2 Heat olive oil in a large nonstick skillet over medium heat. Add garlic and peppers, and cook until soft but not brown, about three minutes.

3 Add drained green beans to pan, toss to combine and heat through. Season with salt and pepper, and serve.

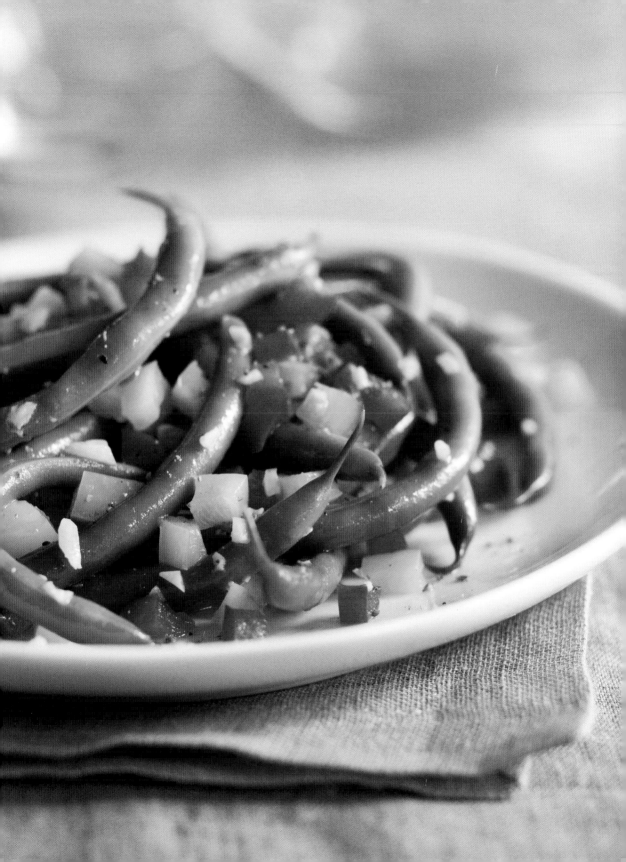

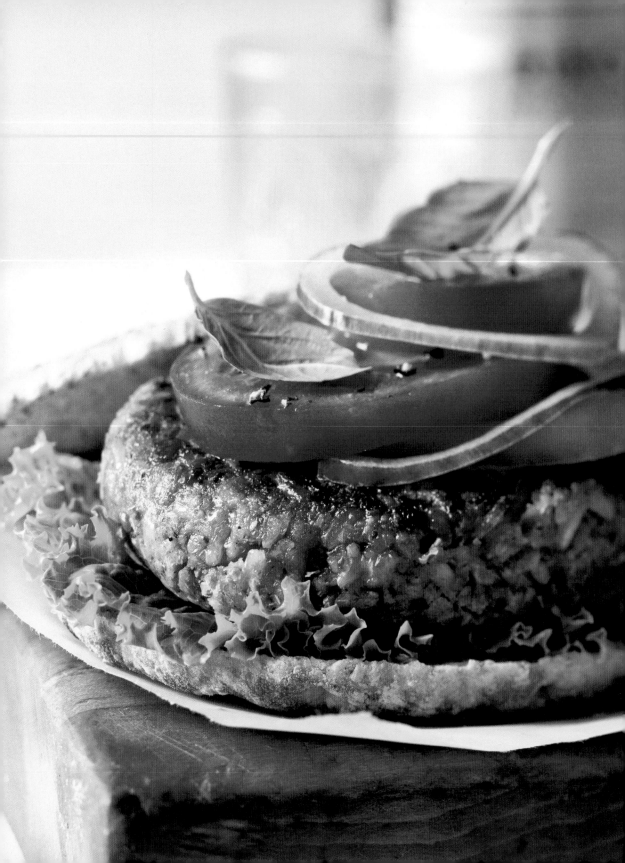

Great Northern White Bean Burgers ⊛

6 servings

PREP: 20 minutes

TOTAL: 26 to 30 minutes

Great Northern beans are white beans that are related to kidney and pinto beans. They don't taste like much on their own, but they easily take on the flavor profiles of spices and herbs. They're also packed with protein and fiber, so you can be confident that this burger will keep you satisfied till your next meal.

Note: This recipe requires pre-cooked brown rice.

✱ If you can't find whole grain breadcrumbs at your local grocery store, make them yourself! Using a cheese grater or food processor, turn whole grain bread or hamburger buns into crumbs. Spread crumbs on a baking sheet and bake at 300°F /150°C until dry, about five to 10 minutes.

Note: Skip the bun if you are following the *Stripped* plan.

Ingredients

1 yellow onion, roughly chopped

1 clove garlic, smashed

1 cup / 240 ml loosely packed parsley

1 cup / 240 ml loosely packed basil

3 Tbsp / 45 ml nutritional yeast

1 Tbsp / 15 ml Dijon mustard

1 egg white

1 tsp / 5 ml garlic powder

1 tsp / 5 ml onion powder

1 tsp / 5 ml chili powder

½ tsp / 2.5 ml celery seed

½ Tbsp / 7.5 ml sea salt

½ tsp / 2.5 ml freshly ground black pepper

1 x 14.5-oz can great Northern white beans, drained and rinsed

1 cup / 240 ml cooked brown rice

½ cup / 120 ml oat bran

2 Tbsp / 30 ml flaxseed meal

1 cup / 240 ml whole grain breadcrumbs✱

Eat-Clean Cooking Spray (see page 214 for recipe)

6 whole grain hamburger buns (optional)

Nutritional Value Per Serving (one patty without bun):

Calories: 216 | Calories from Fat: 20 | Protein: 13.5 g | Carbs: 40 g | Total Fat: 2.5 g | Saturated Fat: 0 g | Trans Fat: 0 g | Fiber: 10 g | Sodium: 578 mg | Cholesterol: 0 mg | Sugar: 2.7 g

Method

1 Add onion, garlic, parsley and basil to a food processor and pulse to combine. Add nutritional yeast, mustard, egg white, garlic powder, onion powder, chili powder, celery seed, salt and pepper, and pulse until finely chopped. Add white beans and pulse until combined, but still chunky.

2 Transfer mixture to a bowl and add brown rice, oat bran, flaxseed meal and breadcrumbs. If mixture is too moist and doesn't easily hold the shape of a patty, add more breadcrumbs until desired consistency is achieved. Shape mixture into six patties, each four inches in diameter.

3 Heat a large nonstick skillet over medium-low heat and coat with Eat-Clean Cooking Spray. Cook patties three to five minutes on each side until browned. For a crispier burger, cook an additional five minutes in a preheated 400°F / 200°C oven or toast in a toaster oven.

4 Serve hot on whole grain buns (skip the bun if you are following the *Stripped* plan) topped with your favorite burger fixings, such as lettuce, tomato, red onion and mustard.

Smack Your Lips Spiced Cauliflower and Tofu over Bulgur Wheat

4 servings
(1½ cups / 360 ml per serving)

PREP: 15 minutes

TOTAL: 30 minutes

Have you ever heard of Meatless Monday? It's an international campaign encouraging people to have one meatless day each week (Monday), to improve both their own health and that of our planet. I serve meatless dishes to my family several times a week – try this one tonight!

Ingredients

¼ tsp / 1.25 ml sea salt

½ cup / 120 ml bulgur wheat

1 tsp / 5 ml olive oil

½ yellow onion, thinly sliced

2 cloves garlic, thinly sliced

1 head cauliflower, cut into bite-sized pieces

8 oz / 227 g reduced fat extra-firm tofu, cut into ½-inch cubes

½ cup / 120 ml golden raisins (optional)

1 tsp / 5 ml ground cumin

½ tsp / 2.5 ml ground coriander

½ tsp / 2.5 ml curry powder

½ tsp / 2.5 ml paprika

¼ tsp / 1.25 ml cayenne

½ tsp / 2.5 ml sea salt

¼ tsp / 1.25 ml freshly ground black pepper

1 cup / 240 ml reduced-sodium vegetable broth

1 bay leaf

¼ cup / 60 ml sliced almonds, divided

¼ cup / 60 ml chopped fresh cilantro

Nutritional Value Per Serving:

Calories: 286 | Calories from Fat: 52 | Protein: 16 g | Carbs: 44 g | Total Fat: 6 g | Saturated Fat: 1 g | Trans Fat: 0 g | Fiber: 8 g | Sodium: 515 mg | Cholesterol: 0 mg | Sugar: 15 g

Method

1 In a small saucepan, bring 1 cup / 240 ml water and salt to boil and stir in bulgur wheat. Cover and reduce heat to simmer for 15 minutes or until all water is absorbed. Remove from heat, fluff, cover and set aside.

2 Heat oil in a large skillet over medium-high heat. Add onion and garlic, and cook until starting to brown, about three minutes. Stir in cauliflower, tofu, raisins (omit if you are following the *Stripped* plan), spices, salt, pepper, vegetable broth and bay leaf.

3 Bring to a boil, cover and reduce heat to simmer until cauliflower is starting to become tender, about three minutes. Uncover and continue to cook until broth reduces by half, about five minutes.

4 Remove from heat and remove bay leaf. Stir in almonds, reserving a few. To serve, top with remaining almonds and cilantro.

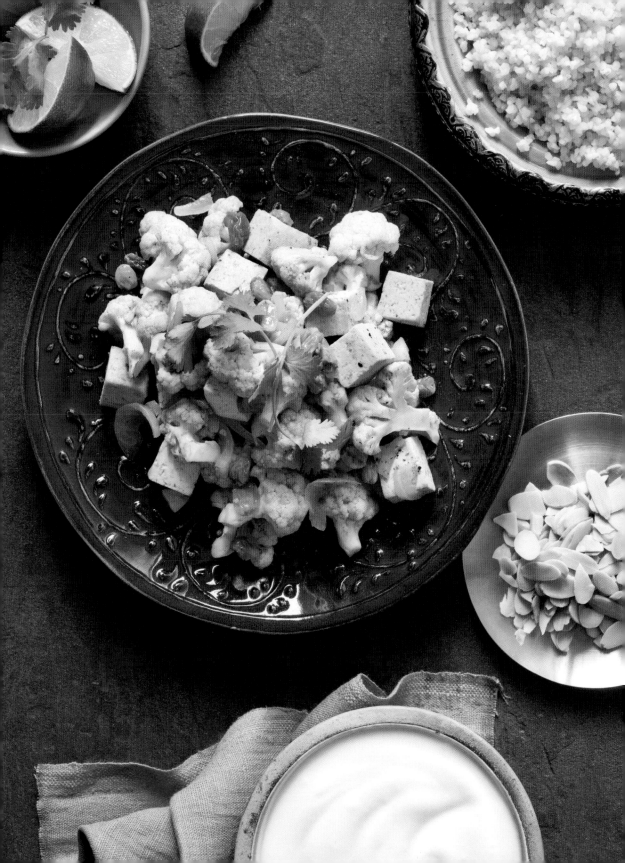

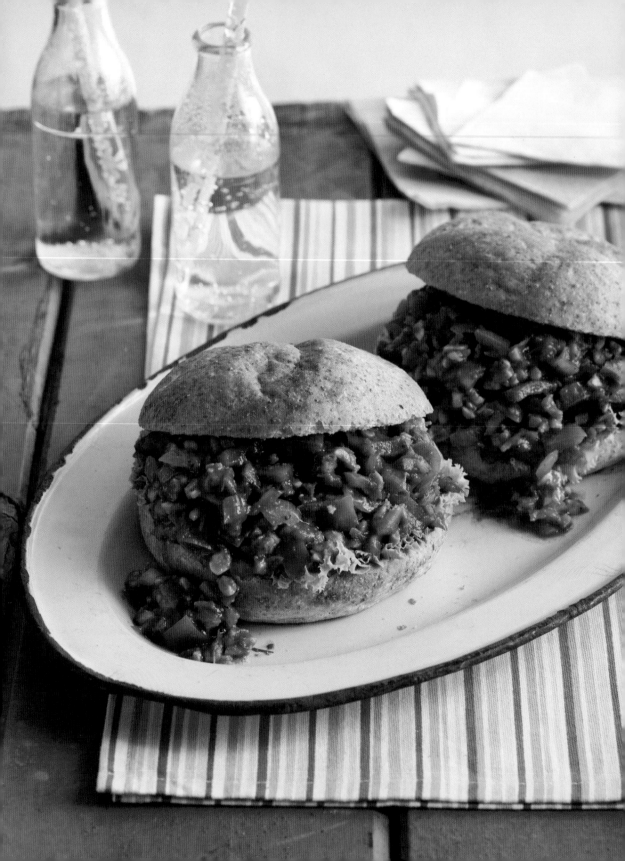

Super Sloppy Janes ⊛

4 servings
(1½ cups / 360 ml per serving)

PREP: 15 minutes

TOTAL: 40 minutes

Sloppy Janes are the feminine version of Sloppy Joes – a loose-meat sandwich traditionally made with ground beef. These Janes are made with tempeh, which is cooked and slightly fermented soy-beans formed into a patty. Tempeh is high in protein and calcium, and it has a textured and nutty flavor.

Ingredients

2 Tbsp / 30 ml yellow mustard

1 Tbsp / 15 ml unsulfured blackstrap molasses

1 Tbsp / 15 ml tomato paste

1 Tbsp / 15 ml unfiltered cider vinegar

1 Tbsp / 15 ml Worcestershire sauce

1 tsp / 5 ml ground cumin

1 tsp / 5 ml chili powder

1 Tbsp / 15 ml olive oil

1 sweet onion, chopped

1 green bell pepper, seeded and chopped

1 carrot, peeled and grated

½ Tbsp / 7.5 ml sea salt

½ tsp / 2.5 ml freshly ground black pepper

8 oz / 227 g organic soy tempeh, crumbled

2 cloves garlic, minced

¼ tsp / 1.25 ml celery seed

1 chipotle pepper in adobo sauce, diced

1 x 14.5-oz can no-salt-added, sugar-free tomato sauce

1 cup / 240 ml low-sodium vegetable broth

4 whole grain buns, split in half (optional)

4 leaves green leaf lettuce

Note: Skip the bun if you are following the *Stripped* plan.

Nutritional Value Per Serving (1 bun, 1 piece lettuce, 1½ cups / 360 ml mixture):

Calories: 350 | Calories from Fat: 81 | Protein: 20 g | Carbs: 52 g | Total Fat: 9 g | Saturated Fat: 1.7 g | Trans Fat: 0 g | Fiber: 14 g | Sodium: 1097 mg | Cholesterol: 0 mg | Sugar: 15 g

Method

1 In a small bowl, mix together mustard, molasses, tomato paste, vinegar, Worcestershire sauce, cumin and chili powder, and set aside.

2 Heat olive oil in a very large nonstick skillet over medium-high heat. Add onion, green pepper, carrot, salt and pepper, and sauté until soft and starting to brown, 10 minutes. Add tempeh, garlic, celery seed and chipotle pepper and cook another three minutes, stirring occasionally.

3 Stir in tomato sauce, vegetable broth and spice mixture (from step one) until combined. Cover and simmer for 10 minutes.

4 Place lettuce on bottom half of bun (skip the bun if you are following the *Stripped* plan) and pile Sloppy Jane mixture on top. Top with other half of bun, put a big napkin on your lap and enjoy!

4 servings
(1 cup / 240 ml per serving)

PREP: 5 minutes

TOTAL: 50 minutes

When the Weather is Frightful, Make Delightful Roasted Butternut Squash Farro Risotto

Risotto is such a comforting classic dish and even more so when butternut squash is involved! I've used farro in this recipe, an ancient grain with a complex, nutty taste. If you've never tried farro, it can be compared to a lighter brown rice.

Ingredients

½ butternut squash

1 Tbsp / 15 ml + ½ tsp / 2.5 ml olive oil, divided

½ tsp / 2.5 ml herbes de Provence

½ cup / 120 ml finely chopped shallots

2 cloves garlic, minced

1 tsp / 5 ml finely chopped fresh thyme

2 tsp / 10 ml finely chopped fresh sage

1 cup / 240 ml farro

4 cups / 960 ml low-sodium chicken or vegetable broth, simmering

1 tsp / 5 ml white-truffle-infused olive oil, to garnish

Sea salt and freshly ground black pepper, to taste

Nutritional Value Per Serving:

Calories: 160 | Calories from Fat: 51 |
Protein: 3.6 g | Carbs: 29 g |
Total Fat: 6 g | Saturated Fat: 1 g |
Trans Fat: 0 g | Fiber: 2 g |
Sodium: 137 mg | Cholesterol: 0 mg |
Sugar: 3 g

Method

1   Preheat oven to 400°F / 200°C. Scoop seeds and pulp from squash. Rub flesh and skin of squash with ½ tsp / 2.5 ml olive oil. Sprinkle flesh with herbes de Provence and season with salt and pepper. Place squash cut side down on a baking sheet and cook in oven until tender when pierced with a knife, about 45 minutes. Set aside to cool.

2   Heat 1 Tbsp / 15 ml olive oil in a large skillet over medium heat. Add shallots, garlic, thyme and sage, and cook for three minutes until soft and fragrant. Stir in farro, season with salt and pepper, and allow to cook for two minutes.

3   Reduce heat to medium-low, stir in ½ cup / 120 ml simmering broth and allow to cook until almost completely absorbed. Continue stirring in ½ cup / 120 ml broth at a time, allowing liquid to absorb before adding more until farro is tender, but still slightly chewy, 30 to 35 minutes.

4   Scrape cooled squash into a bowl and mash. Stir into risotto. Taste and make any final adjustments to seasoning with salt and pepper. Spoon risotto into shallow bowls and top with truffle oil.

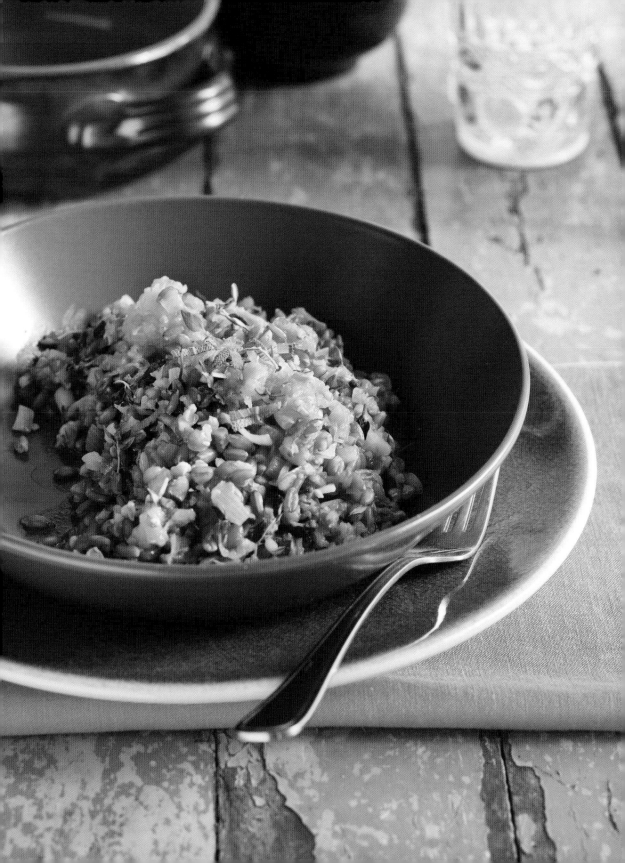

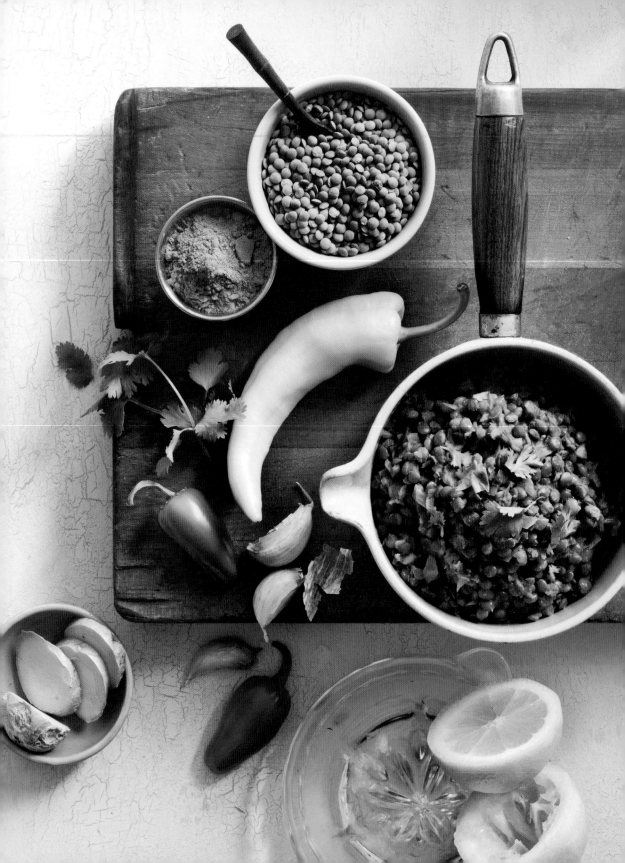

Hello Lentil Dal-ly

4 servings
(1 cup / 240 ml per serving)

PREP: 10 minutes

TOTAL: 70 to 85 minutes

Dal is a spicy Indian soup made up of lentils and pulsed vegetables. It's a perfect vegetarian dish for a weeknight, because it's chock full of protein and easy to make. Eat it on its own or serve over brown rice or vegetables.

Ingredients

3 cloves garlic, smashed

1 piece fresh ginger about the size of a large thumb, peeled and roughly chopped

1 onion, roughly chopped

1 green pepper, seeded and roughly chopped

1 banana pepper, seeded and roughly chopped

1 jalapeno, seeds removed and roughly chopped (for a spicier dish, leave seeds in)

1 tsp / 5 ml olive oil

2 tsp / 10 ml turmeric

1 tsp / 5 ml cumin

½ Tbsp / 7.5 ml sea salt

½ tsp / 2.5 ml freshly ground black pepper

1 cup / 240 ml rinsed and drained brown lentils

Juice of 1 lemon (2 to 3 Tbsp / 30 to 45 ml)

½ cup / 120 ml Yogurt Cheese to garnish (optional, see page 301 for recipe)

¼ cup / 60 ml chopped cilantro (optional)

Nutritional Value Per Serving (without Yogurt Cheese and cilantro):

Calories: 214 | Calories from Fat: 18 | Protein: 13 g | Carbs: 37 g | Total Fat: 1.7 g | Saturated Fat: 0 g | Trans Fat: 0 g | Fiber: 16 g | Sodium: 621 mg | Cholesterol: 0 mg | Sugar: 3.5 g

Method

1 In a food processor, pulse garlic, ginger, onion, peppers and jalapeno until finely chopped.

2 Heat olive oil in a medium pot over medium-high heat. Add processed vegetables, turmeric, cumin, salt and pepper. Cook until vegetables are soft, but not browned, about three minutes. Stir in lentils and three-and-a-half cups / 840 ml water. Bring to a boil, cover, reduce heat to low and simmer, stirring occasionally, one hour and 15 minutes. Uncover and remove from heat.

3 Using a potato masher, mash lentils until mostly smooth. Stir in lemon juice and serve. Top each serving with 2 Tbsp / 30 ml Yogurt Cheese (omit if you are following the *Stripped* plan) and 1 Tbsp / 15 ml cilantro, if desired.

Surfer Dude Fish Tacos with Tomatillo Salsa Verde ⊕

4 servings
(2 tacos per serving)

PREP: 20 minutes

TOTAL: 27 minutes

The first fish tacos were found in Baja California in Mexico. This makes sense to me as they are a delightful blend of American and Mexican cuisines. In the Southern United States, you can find fish-taco street vendors. (I guarantee these are healthier and will taste better!)

Ingredients

TOMATILLO SALSA VERDE:

½ lb / 227 g tomatillos, skins removed and quartered

½ yellow onion, cut into quarters

1 jalapeno, quartered, seeds and ribs removed

1 clove garlic, smashed

½ cup / 120 ml roughly chopped cilantro

½ cup / 120 ml low-sodium vegetable broth

Juice of ½ lime (1 to 2 Tbsp / 15 to 30 ml)

½ tsp / 2.5 ml sea salt

¼ tsp / 1.25 ml freshly ground black pepper

FISH TACOS:

Eat-Clean Cooking Spray (see page 214 for recipe)

1 lb / 454 g true cod, pin bones removed

½ tsp / 2.5 ml ground cumin

¼ tsp / 1.25 ml sea salt

⅛ tsp / pinch freshly ground black pepper

8 whole grain sprouted corn tortillas, warmed

¼ head green cabbage, shredded

¼ head red cabbage, shredded

1 tomato, diced

1 avocado, sliced

Yogurt Cheese to garnish (optional, see page 301 for recipe)

Cilantro, to garnish

1 lime, cut into wedges, to garnish

Note: Skip the tortillas if you are following the *Stripped* plan.

Nutritional Value Per Serving:

Calories: 408 | Calories from Fat: 92 | Protein: 33 g | Carbs: 49 g | Total Fat: 11 g | Saturated Fat: 1.25 g | Trans Fat: 0 g | Fiber: 12 g | Sodium: 579 mg | Cholesterol: 54 mg | Sugar: 9.8 g

Method

1 Heat a dry cast iron skillet over medium-high heat. Add tomatillos, onion, jalapeno and garlic and cook until charred and slightly soft, three minutes. Pour charred ingredients into blender and add cilantro, broth, lime juice, salt and pepper. Blend until smooth. Set aside.

2 Heat a large skillet over medium-high heat and coat with Eat-Clean Cooking Spray. Slice cod into one-inch strips and season with cumin, salt and pepper. Place cod in skillet in a single layer and cook two minutes on each side until opaque.

3 To build the tacos, place fish in warmed tortillas (omit if following the *Stripped* plan), top with green and red cabbage, tomato, avocado and Yogurt Cheese (omit if following the *Stripped* plan), and generously spoon Tomatillo Salsa Verde over top. Garnish with cilantro and lime juice. Serve immediately.

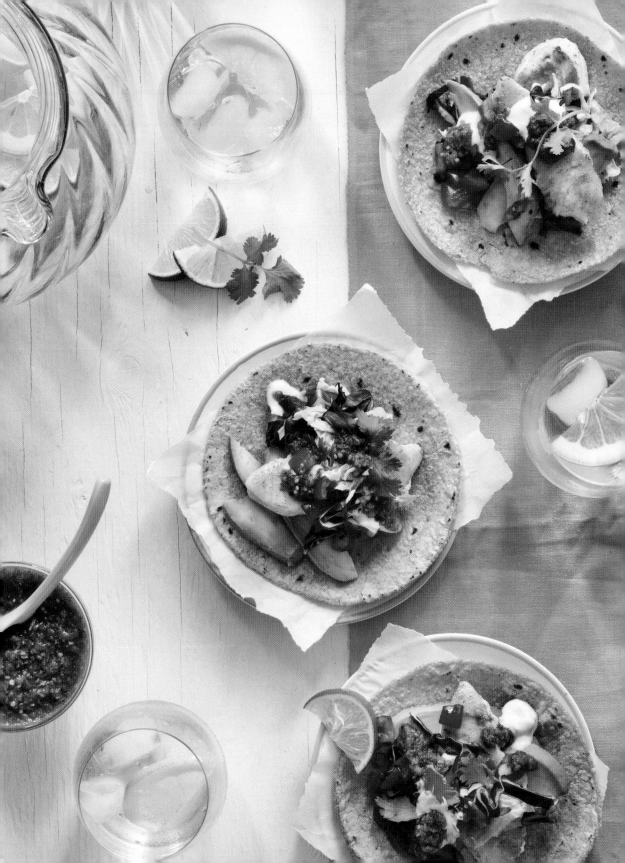

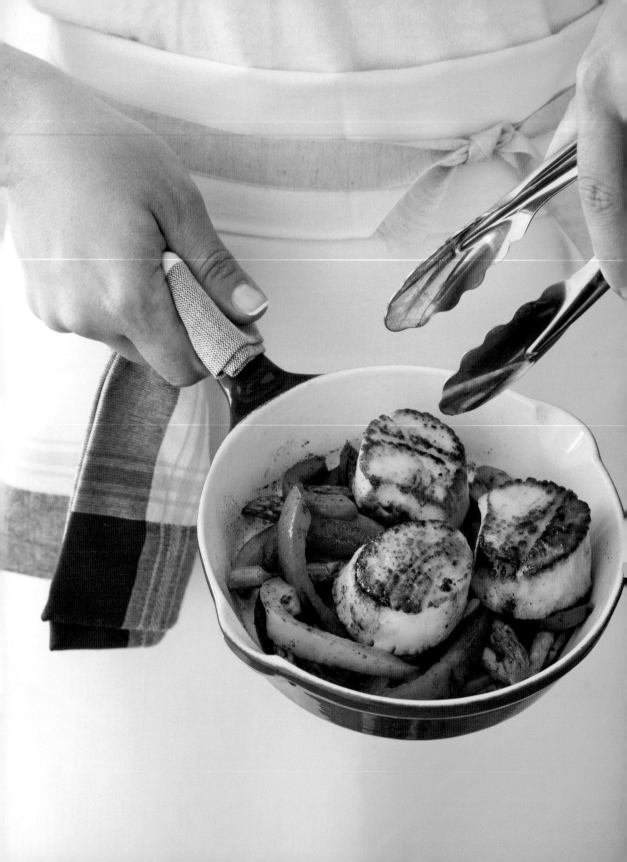

Scallops a la Plancha with Sautéed Asparagus and Peppers

"A la Plancha" is Spanish for "grilled on a metal plate." The cooking method for this recipe – cooking dry scallops on a dry skillet without any oil – really brings out the natural flavor of the mollusks. Enjoy!

Ingredients

1 lb / 454 g wild caught large scallops

⅛ tsp / pinch sea salt

⅛ tsp / pinch freshly ground black pepper

1 tsp / 5 ml olive oil

1 red pepper, seeded and thinly sliced

1 yellow or orange pepper, seeded and thinly sliced

2 cups / 480 ml baby asparagus, sliced into 3-inch-long pieces (match length of sliced peppers)

¼ tsp / 1.25 ml ground cumin

¼ tsp / 1.25 ml paprika

¼ tsp / 1.25 ml turmeric

¼ tsp / 1.25 ml onion powder

Nutritional Value Per Serving:

Calories: 143 | Calories from Fat: 22 | Protein: 21 g | Carbs: 9.5 g | Total Fat: 2.5 g | Saturated Fat: 0 g | Trans Fat: 0 g | Fiber: 2.4 g | Sodium: 232 mg | Cholesterol: 37 mg | Sugar: 2.5 g

Method

1 Heat a large cast iron skillet over high heat. Make sure scallops are dry, then season with a pinch of salt and pepper. Add scallops to dry skillet, turn heat down to medium and cook two minutes on each side until slightly charred and tender. Remove and set aside.

2 Return skillet to stove and add olive oil. Add peppers, asparagus, cumin, paprika, turmeric and onion powder. Season with a pinch of salt and pepper, and sauté until tender-crisp, three minutes.

3 Divide vegetables equally among four plates and top with scallops.

Wild Boar Sugo ⍟

6 servings
(1¹⁄₃ cups / 320 ml per servings)

PREP: 15 minutes

TOTAL: 135 minutes

Sugo, similar to ragu, is a long-simmered pasta sauce that works well over pasta, grains and vegetables. This version is made with boar meat, a flavorful alternative to pork.

Ingredients

2 tsp / 10 ml olive oil, divided

1 lb / 454 g lean boar stew meat, trimmed of extra fat and cut into 1-inch chunks

1½ tsp / 7.5 ml sea salt, divided

¾ tsp / 3.75 ml freshly ground black pepper, divided

1 medium yellow onion, diced

2 carrots, diced

2 ribs celery, diced

1 Tbsp / 15 ml chopped fresh oregano or marjoram

1 Tbsp / 15 ml chopped fresh sage

1 Tbsp / 15 ml chopped fresh thyme

2 cloves garlic, chopped

½ tsp / 2.5 ml crushed red pepper flakes

¼ tsp / 1.25 ml allspice

1 x 14.5-oz can no-salt-added diced tomatoes

1 x 14.5-oz can no-salt-added, sugar-free tomato sauce

½ to 1 cup / 120 to 240 ml low-sodium chicken broth, or enough to completely cover pork

Note: Skip the optional noodles if you are following the *Stripped* plan.

Nutritional Value Per Serving:

Calories: 167 | Calories from Fat: 39 | Protein: 18 g | Carbs: 14 g | Total Fat: 4 g | Saturated Fat: 1 g | Trans Fat: 0 g | Fiber: 4 g | Sodium: 644 mg | Cholesterol: 56mg | Sugar: 8 g

Method

1 Preheat the oven to 275°F / 135°C. Heat 1 tsp / 5 ml olive oil in a large ovenproof pot or Dutch oven over high heat on the stove. Pat boar dry with a paper towel and add to pot in a single layer, being careful not to overcrowd. Season with ½ tsp / 2.5 ml salt and ¼ tsp / 1.25 ml pepper. Let boar brown, about three minutes. Remove to a bowl and set aside.

2 Reduce heat to medium and add remaining 1 tsp / 5 ml olive oil, onion, carrots, celery, oregano, sage and thyme. Season with remaining 1 tsp / 5 ml salt and ½ tsp / 2.5 ml pepper, and sauté until softened and starting to brown, about three minutes. Stir in garlic, red pepper flakes and allspice, and cook for one minute longer.

3 Stir in diced tomatoes and tomato sauce and scrape bottom of pot to loosen any crusty bits. Add boar and any accumulated juices back into pot, and then add chicken broth. Bring liquid to a boil, cover and place in oven to slowly cook until tender, about two-and-a-half hours. Boar is done when fork tender and almost falling apart.

4 Remove from oven and using a potato masher, break up boar and vegetables. Sugo will be chunky. Taste, and make any final adjustments to seasoning with sea salt and freshly ground black pepper.

5 Serve over your favorite whole grain, whole wheat pasta (skip if you are following the *Stripped* plan) or steamed vegetables.

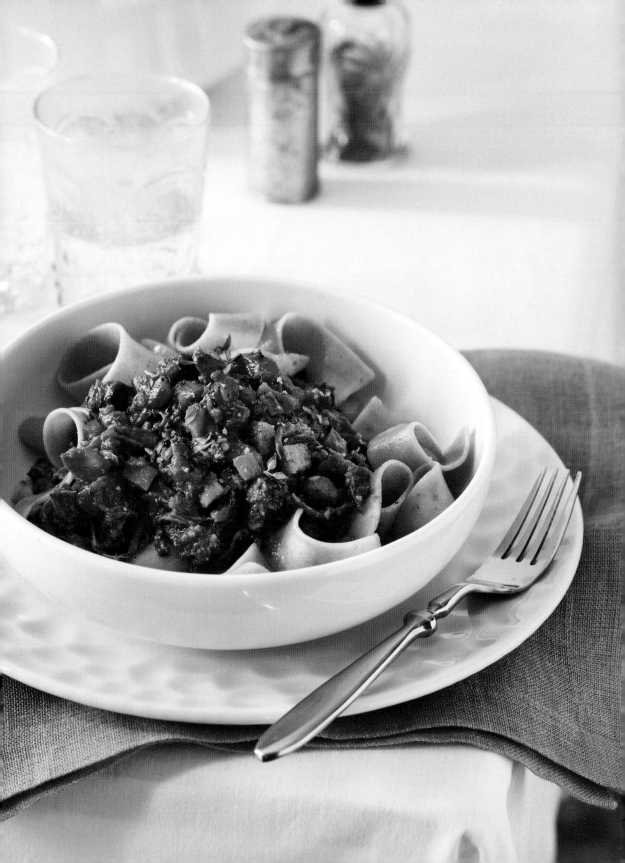

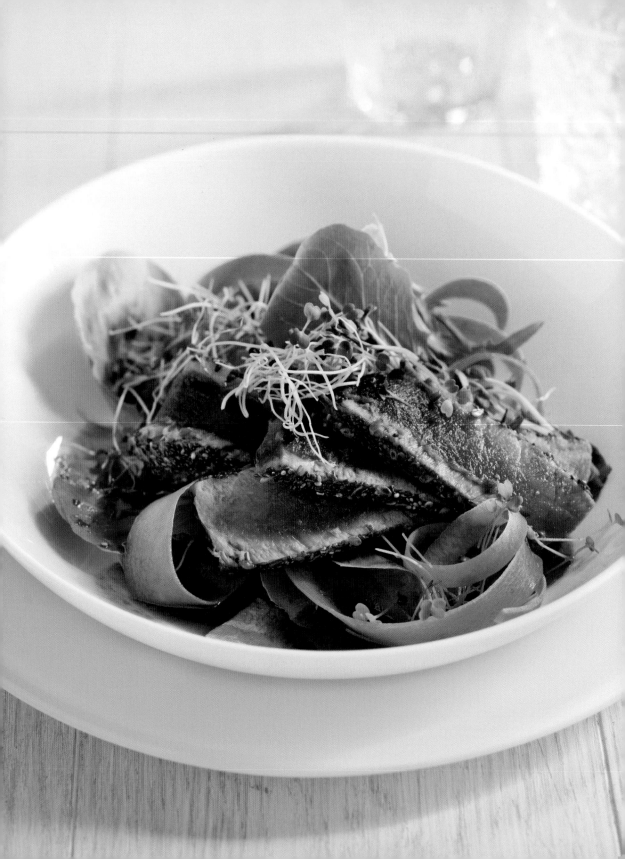

You'll Feel Like a Super Hero Super Seed Seared Tuna with Microgreens

Microgreens are tiny edible greens with surprisingly intense flavors produced from the seeds of vegetables, herbs and other plants. Combined with the healthy fats found in flaxseed and chia seeds, this dish is a superfoods powerhouse.

Ingredients

DRESSING:

2 Tbsp / 30 ml reduced-sodium soy sauce

2 tsp / 10 ml toasted sesame oil

¼ tsp / 1.25 ml sambal oelek (ground fresh chili paste)

1 tsp / 5 ml rice vinegar

SALAD:

4 cups / 960 ml mixed baby greens

1 cup / 240 ml microgreens (such as daikon radish, red rose radish, broccoli, sunflower)

1 carrot

TUNA:

2 Tbsp / 30 ml roasted golden flaxseed

2 Tbsp / 30 ml chia seeds

Eat-Clean Cooking Spray (see page 214 for recipe)

2 x 8 oz / 454 g pieces good-quality ahi tuna (sashimi grade recommended)

Sea salt and freshly ground black pepper

Nutritional Value Per Serving:

Calories: 225 | Calories from Fat: 60 | Protein: 38 g | Carbs: 8 g | Total Fat: 6.4 g | Saturated Fat: 0.6 g | Trans Fat: 0 g | Fiber: 5 g | Sodium: 404 mg | Cholesterol: 60 mg | Sugar: 2 g

Method

1   Whisk together all dressing ingredients and set aside.

2   In a bowl, add baby greens and microgreens. Using a serrated peeler, peel carrot and discard peelings. Place carrot on a flat surface and using peeler, peel thin strips down carrot (they will look like ribbons). Add carrot ribbons to greens, gently toss and set aside.

3   Combine flaxseed and chia seeds in a bowl. Heat a large nonstick skillet over medium-high heat and spray with Eat-Clean Cooking Spray. Lightly season ahi on all sides with salt and pepper. Place ahi in seed bowl and evenly coat all sides with seeds. Place ahi in skillet and sear for two minutes on each side. Remove to a cutting board and let rest for five minutes.

4   To serve, divide salad among four plates. Thinly slice tuna and fan out next to salad. Drizzle salad and tuna with dressing and top with more microgreens, if desired.

4 servings

PREP: 20 minutes

TOTAL: 40 minutes

Saigon Fusion Noodle Bowl with Grilled Chicken ⊕

Japanese buckwheat noodles, also known as soba noodles, are thin brown noodles made from buckwheat flour. In Japan, they slurp these noodles noisily, as it is considered polite. They are also quite common as a housewarming present. Fascinating!

Note: Skip the noodles if you are following the *Stripped* plan.

Nutritional Value Per Serving:

Calories: 304 | Calories from Fat: 48 | Protein: 32 g | Carbs: 31 g | Total Fat: 5 g | Saturated Fat: 0.5 g | Trans Fat: 0 g | Fiber: 4 g | Sodium: 555 mg | Cholesterol: 65 mg | Sugar: 4 g

Ingredients

NOODLE BOWL:

4 oz Japanese-style buckwheat noodles (optional)

Eat-Clean Cooking Spray (see page 214 for recipe)

16 oz / 454 g chicken breast

Sea salt and freshly ground black pepper, to taste

1 tsp / 5 ml safflower oil

½ red pepper, seeded and sliced

½ yellow or orange pepper, seeded and sliced

2 cups / 480 ml shredded cabbage, green or red or both

¼ yellow onion, thinly sliced

2 stalks celery, sliced diagonally

2 cups / 480 ml white button mushrooms, sliced

2 cloves garlic, minced

½ tsp / 2.5 ml sesame oil

1 Tbsp / 15 ml low-sodium tamari

3 cups / 720 ml thinly sliced green leaf lettuce

¼ English cucumber, thinly sliced into half moons

¼ cup / 60 ml thinly sliced scallions

1 tsp / 5 ml golden roasted whole flaxseed

Cilantro, to garnish

DRESSING:

3 Tbsp / 45 ml rice vinegar

½ tsp / 2.5 ml Asian fish sauce

½ tsp / 2.5 ml sambal oelek (ground fresh chili paste)

1 tsp / 5 ml sesame oil

Method

NOODLE BOWL:

1 Bring a medium pot of water to boil over high heat. Cook buckwheat noodles according to package directions (omit if following the *Stripped* plan). Drain and set aside.

2 Heat a grill or grill pan to medium-high heat and spray with Eat-Clean Cooking Spray, if necessary. Season both sides of chicken with salt and pepper, and cook four to five minutes on each side until done. Remove chicken from heat and set aside.

3 Heat safflower oil in a large nonstick skillet over medium-high heat. Add peppers, cabbage, onion, celery, mushrooms and garlic. Season with salt and pepper and sauté until soft and starting to brown, about five minutes. Stir in sesame oil and tamari. Remove vegetables from heat and set aside.

4 In a large serving bowl, place lettuce, then noodles (if using) and sautéed vegetables. Thinly slice cooked chicken on the diagonal and fan out on top of vegetables. Add cucumbers around chicken, sprinkle with scallions and flaxseed, and garnish with a few sprigs of fresh cilantro. Serve with dressing on the side to pour over salad at the table.

DRESSING:

1 In a small bowl, whisk together all dressing ingredients until thoroughly combined.

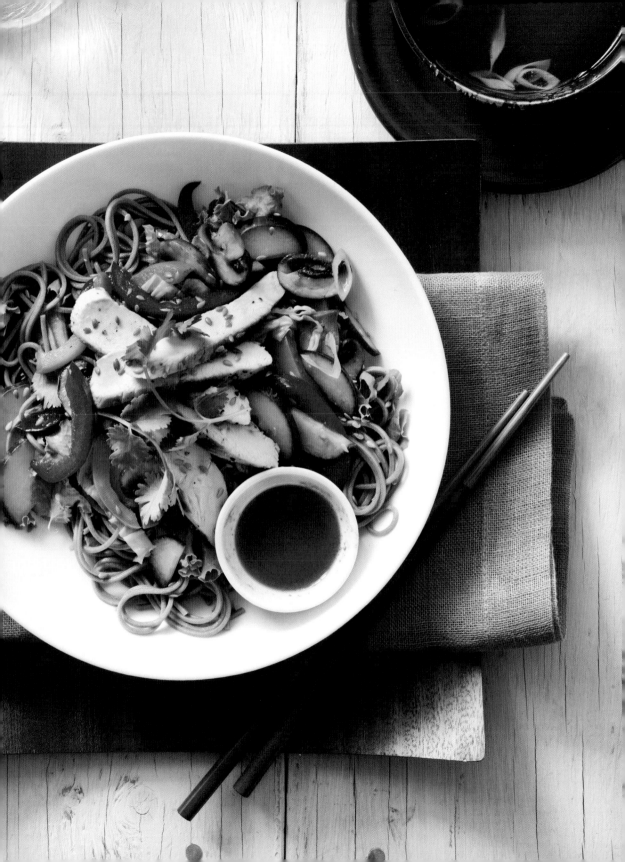

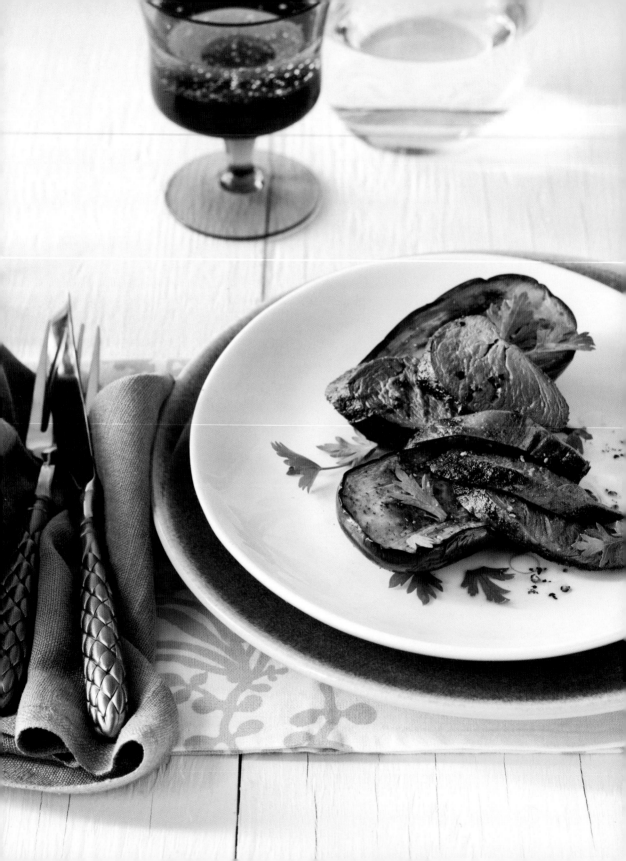

Chinese Five Spice Venison with Indian Eggplant

4 servings

PREP: 10 minutes

TOTAL: 35 to 40 minutes

If you've never tried venison, now is the time! It's a tender meat with a velvety texture and cooked right, you'd never guess it's so low in fat. Inspired by the many flavors of the world, this easy-to-make exotic dish will send your taste buds on a trip around the globe.

Ingredients

1 lb / 454 g (about 6 cups / 1440 ml) Indian eggplant, cut in half lengthwise

Eat-Clean Cooking Spray (see page 214 for recipe)

⅛ tsp / pinch cayenne pepper

1 tsp / 5 ml sea salt, divided

½ tsp / 2.5 ml freshly ground black pepper, divided

2 Tbsp / 30 ml chopped fresh flat leaf parsley

½ tsp / 2.5 ml Chinese five spice powder

½ tsp / 2.5 ml ground cumin

¼ tsp / 1.25 ml garlic powder

1 lb / 454 g venison tenderloin

1 tsp / 5 ml olive oil

Nutritional Value Per Serving:

Calories: 210 | Calories from Fat: 35 | Protein: 34 g | Carbs: 8.6 g | Total Fat: 3.6 g | Saturated Fat: 1.4 g | Trans Fat: 0g | Fiber: 4 g | Sodium: 672 mg | Cholesterol: 100 mg | Sugar: 4 g

Method

1　Preheat oven to 400°F / 200°C. Place eggplant in a single layer on a baking sheet and coat with Eat-Clean Cooking Spray. Sprinkle eggplant with cayenne, ½ tsp / 2.5 ml salt and ¼ tsp / 1.25 ml pepper; roast for 15 minutes. Remove from oven, flip eggplant, coat with more cooking spray and continue roasting until soft and lightly browned, 10 to 15 minutes. Remove to a bowl and toss with parsley. Set aside.

2　In a separate small bowl, combine Chinese five spice powder, cumin, garlic powder, and remaining ½ tsp / 2.5 ml salt and ¼ tsp / 1.25 ml pepper. Coat venison tenderloin evenly on all sides with spice mixture, rubbing and patting it in.

3　Heat olive oil in an ovenproof skillet over medium-high heat. Once hot, add venison and cook without disturbing until browned, two to three minutes. Turn venison over and place skillet in preheated oven to cook until desired doneness, five to seven minutes for medium rare.

4　Remove venison to a cutting board to rest for five minutes. Thinly slice and serve with roasted eggplant.

Stir-Fried Ginger Beef with Snap Peas, Shiitake Mushrooms and Red Peppers

4 servings

PREP: 20 minutes

TOTAL: 25 to 26 minutes

Make sure to have all your ingredients chopped and prepared before you start, use a hot wok with cold oil, and make sure your meats and vegetables are dry before you start cooking – this way they'll stir-fry, not braise, and you'll have browned meat and tender-crisp veggies.

Nutritional Value Per Serving:

Calories: 238 | Calories from Fat: 106 | Protein: 20 g | Carbs: 11 g | Total Fat: 12 g | Saturated Fat: 3 g | Trans Fat: 0 g | Fiber: 3 g | Sodium: 526 mg | Cholesterol: 42 mg | Sugar: 3.6 g

Ingredients

12 oz / 340 g lean flank steak, cut across the grain into 2-inch long strips, ¼-inch thick

1 Tbsp / 15 ml + 2 tsp / 10 ml minced fresh ginger, divided

2 tsp / 10 ml reduced-sodium tamari, divided

2 tsp / 10 ml rice vinegar, divided

1 tsp / 5 ml sambal oelek (ground fresh chili paste)

1 tsp / 5 ml sesame oil

1 tsp / 5 ml arrowroot

¾ tsp / 3.75 ml sea salt, divided

¼ tsp / 1.25 ml freshly ground black pepper

3 tsp / 15 ml grapeseed oil, divided

4 green onions, halved lengthwise and cut into 2-inch pieces

1 red pepper, seeds and core removed, thinly sliced

1 baby yellow squash, halved lengthwise and cut into half moons ¼-inch thick

1 clove garlic, minced

8 oz / 227 g shiitake mushrooms, stems removed and caps quartered

1 Tbsp / 15 ml low-sodium broth (beef, chicken, or vegetable), or water

8 oz / 227 g sugar snap peas, strings removed

1 Tbsp / 15 ml golden roasted flaxseed

Method

1 In a medium bowl, combine steak, 1 Tbsp / 15 ml ginger, 1 tsp / 5 ml tamari, 1 tsp / 5 ml rice vinegar, sambal oelek, sesame oil, arrowroot, ¼ tsp / 1.25 ml salt and ¼ tsp / 1.25 ml pepper. Stir to mix.

2 Heat a 14-inch flat-bottomed wok or 12-inch skillet over high heat until a drop of water will vaporize in a second of contact. Swirl in 1 tsp / 5 ml grapeseed oil, add steak and spread evenly in one layer to cook without moving for one minute. Then, using metal tongs or a metal spatula, stir-fry for one minute until steak is lightly browned but not yet cooked through. Add green onions and stir-fry another 30 seconds until steak is cooked through. Remove to a large bowl and set aside.

3 Return wok to stove over high heat until hot enough to vaporize a drop of water. Swirl in 1 tsp / 5 ml grapeseed oil, add 1 tsp / 5 ml ginger, red pepper, squash and ¼ tsp / 1.25 ml salt. Stir-fry one to two minutes until vegetables are slightly softened. Remove to bowl with steak and set aside.

4 Return wok to stove over high heat until hot enough to vaporize a drop of water. Swirl in 1 tsp / 5 ml grapeseed oil, add remaining 1 tsp / 5 ml ginger, garlic and shiitake mushrooms, and stir-fry 30 seconds. Add remaining 1 tsp / 5 ml tamari and 1 tsp / 5 ml rice vinegar and broth. Cover and cook 30 seconds until almost all liquid is absorbed. Add snap peas and ¼ tsp / 1.25 ml salt and stir-fry one minute until peas turn bright green. Remove to bowl with steak and veggies.

5 Toss steak and veggies to combine. To serve, top with flaxseed and serve with quinoa or brown rice.

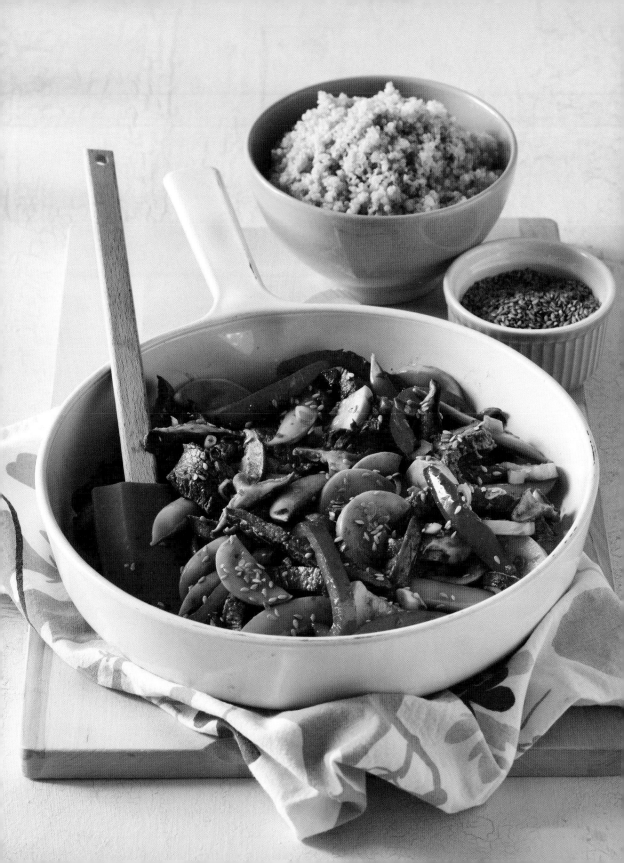

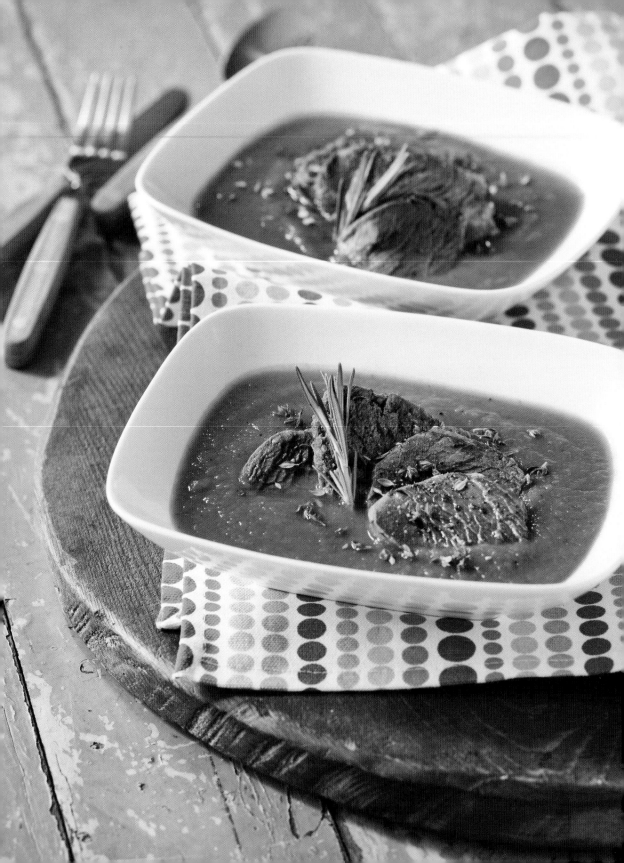

Not Your Mom's Elk Pot Roast with Root Vegetable Sauce

6 servings
(⅙ roast and ⅔ cup / 160 ml sauce per serving)

PREP: 10 minutes

TOTAL: 250 minutes

Love pot roast but hate eating so much fatty beef? Try elk – it's a low-fat, high-protein alternative to beef and it tastes delicious. This recipe makes four cups of Root Vegetable Sauce, so you'll have some left over. Try it as a soup for tomorrow's lunch!

Ingredients

3 tsp / 15 ml olive oil, divided

1½ to 2 lbs / 681 to 908 g elk shoulder roast

2 tsp / 10 ml sea salt, divided

1 tsp / 5 ml freshly ground black pepper, divided

1 medium yellow onion, chopped

2 carrots, chopped

2 stalks celery, chopped

2 parsnips, chopped

1 Tbsp / 15 ml chopped fresh thyme

1 tsp / 5 ml chopped fresh rosemary

2 cloves garlic, smashed

¼ tsp / 1.25 ml ground cloves

2 cups / 480 ml low-sodium beef broth

1 bay leaf

Nutritional Value Per Serving:

Calories: 245 | Calories from Fat: 41 | Protein: 37 g | Carbs: 13 g | Total Fat: 4.7 g | Saturated Fat: 1 g | Trans Fat: 0 g | Fiber: 3.6 g | Sodium: 786 mg | Cholesterol: 82 mg | Sugar: 4.5 g

Method

1 Preheat oven to 275°F / 135°C. Heat 2 tsp / 10 ml olive oil in an oven-safe braising pot or Dutch oven over high heat. Make sure roast is dry, then season on all sides with 1 tsp / 5 ml salt and ½ tsp / 2.5 ml pepper, and place in the pot. Brown on all sides, then remove and set aside.

2 Reduce heat to medium and add remaining 1 tsp / 5 ml olive oil. Add onion, carrots, celery, parsnips, thyme, rosemary, garlic, cloves and remaining 1 tsp / 5 ml salt and ½ tsp / 2.5 ml pepper. Sauté until soft and starting to brown, about three minutes. Add broth and bay leaf, and scrape brown bits off bottom of pot. Place roast back in pot, nestling it among the vegetables, making sure that broth comes almost halfway up side of roast.

3 Bring to a boil then cover and place in oven to cook until roast is fork tender and will easily break apart, about four hours. Transfer cooked roast to a cutting board and cover to keep warm.

4 Remove bay leaf from pot and discard. Using a blender, blend liquid and vegetables until very smooth, working in batches if necessary (be careful when blending hot liquids because they can expand). Taste sauce and make any adjustments to seasoning with salt and pepper.

5 Serve roast with vegetable purée.

Salmon with Sweet 'n' Tangy Pineapple Chutney

4 servings

PREP: 15 minutes

TOTAL: 35 minutes

The word chutney comes from the East Indian word "chatni," which refers to crushing and literally means, "to make chutney." This pineapple chutney is different from the thick, jam-like chutneys popular in Indian cuisine, but works wonderfully with any grilled meat.

Nutritional Value Per Serving:
Calories: 328 | Calories from Fat: 106 | Protein: 31 g | Carbs: 19 g | Total Fat: 14 g | Saturated Fat: 2 g | Trans Fat: 0 g | Fiber: 2 g | Sodium: 363 mg | Cholesterol: 87 mg | Sugar: 14.5 g

Ingredients

SALMON:
1 tsp / 5 ml extra virgin olive oil
4 x 5 oz wild-caught salmon fillets, skin and pin bones removed
½ tsp / 2.5 ml sea salt
¼ tsp / 1.25 ml freshly ground black pepper

CHUTNEY:
1 orange
1 x 8-oz can pineapple tidbits with juice
1 red pepper, seeds and core removed, diced
½ red onion, diced
1 jalapeno, seeds and core removed, minced
1 clove garlic, thinly sliced

1 tsp / 5 ml grated fresh ginger
Juice of 1 lime (2 to 3 Tbsp / 30 to 45 ml)
1 Tbsp / 15 ml unfiltered cider vinegar
¼ tsp / 1.25 ml sea salt
¼ tsp / 1.25 ml freshly ground black pepper
1 tsp / 5 ml arrowroot

Method

SALMON:

1 Heat 1 tsp / 5 ml oil in a large nonstick skillet over medium-high heat. Season both sides of salmon with salt and pepper. Place salmon presentation side (side that did not have skin) down in the pan. Cook until lightly browned, flip, and continue cooking until done, about six minutes total. Salmon will be almost completely opaque and will gently flake apart when a knife is inserted into the thickest part of the fish.

2 Serve salmon topped with chutney (method directly below).

CHUTNEY:

1 Zest half orange into a small saucepan. Cut a quarter-inch off top and bottom of orange so that it can stand upright on a cutting board. Cut away remaining peel and pith, working from top to bottom, and discard. Segment orange, cutting between membranes. Cut each segment in half and add to saucepan. Squeeze juice from remaining membrane into saucepan and discard membrane.

2 Add the rest of the chutney ingredients to saucepan, up to and including black pepper. Place on stove over medium-high heat. Bring to a boil then reduce heat to simmer until chutney is soft and flavors combine, stirring occasionally, about 20 minutes. In a small bowl, mix arrowroot with 1 tsp / 5 ml water and stir into chutney. Increase heat to simmer for one minute until chutney liquid thickens slightly. Remove from heat and set aside to cool slightly.

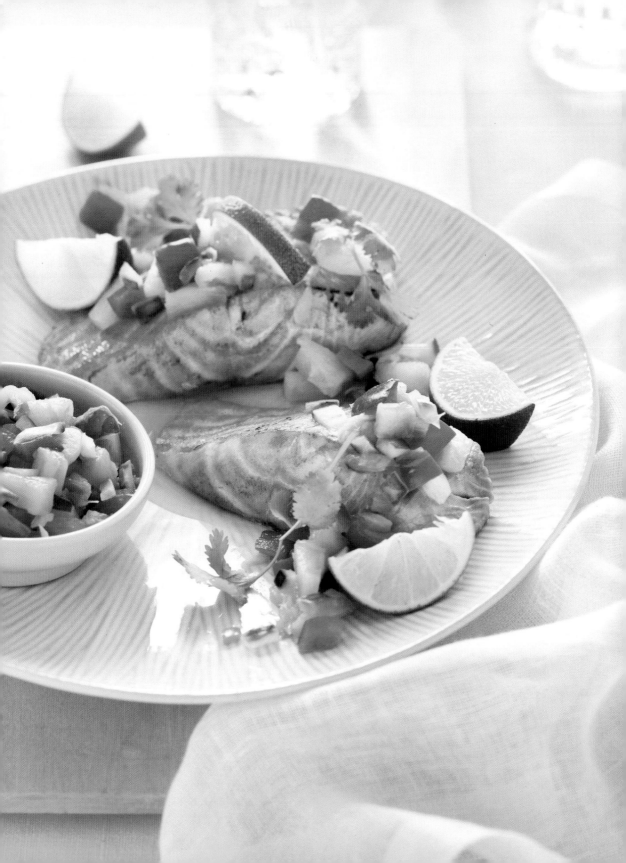

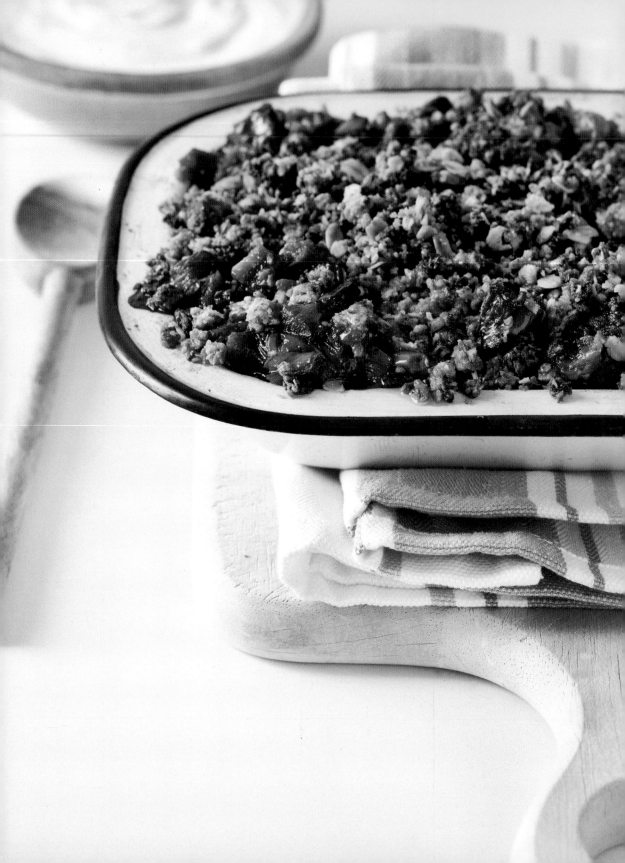

Everybody Loves Rhubarb Flax Crisp ✪

6 servings
(½ cup / 120 ml per serving)

PREP: 15 minutes

TOTAL: 65 to 75 minutes

Rhubarb is a fruit and its stalks are revered for their sweet and tart flavor, which is perfect for pies, jam and other desserts. Here I've combined rhubarb's sweetness with the goodness of flaxseed and coconut oil, two healthy fats that keep your motor running in top condition. Dessert can be good for you!

Ingredients

FILLING:
4 cups / 960 ml diced rhubarb
Juice of 1 orange
   (about ¼ cup / 60 ml)
1 Tbsp / 15 ml arrowroot powder
3 Tbsp / 45 ml honey

TOPPING:
½ cup / 120 ml pitted dates
½ cup / 120 ml whole wheat flour
½ cup / 120 ml whole oats
2 Tbsp / 30 ml flaxseed meal, or
   ground flaxseed
½ tsp / 2.5 ml cinnamon
¼ tsp / 1.25 ml nutmeg
⅛ tsp / pinch sea salt
1 Tbsp / 15 ml honey
3 Tbsp / 45 ml virgin coconut oil,
   softened

Note: This dish is a treat and is not part of your 28-day plan to get *Stripped*.

Nutritional Value Per Serving:

Calories: 235 | Calories from Fat: 75 | Protein: 3.6 g | Carbs: 33 g | Total Fat: 8.6 g | Saturated Fat: 6.6 g | Trans Fat: 0 g | Fiber: 4.8 g | Sodium: 45 mg | Cholesterol: 0 mg | Sugar: 21 g

Method

1 Preheat oven to 350°F / 175°C. In a medium bowl, combine rhubarb, orange juice, arrowroot and honey. Pour into a baking dish.

2 In a food processor, pulse dates into small pieces. Add rest of topping ingredients and pulse to combine. The topping should be moist enough to stick together when pressed between your fingers. Pour topping onto rhubarb mixture.

3 Place dish on a baking sheet to catch any spills. Bake for 50 to 60 minutes until bubbling. Serve warm.

Satisfy the Craving with Clean Chocolate Cupcakes ⓧ

14 servings

PREP: 15 minutes

TOTAL: 35 to 40 minutes

Let's face it – without cupcakes, life just wouldn't be worth living! Check out the ingredients list for these babies ... no sugar! They are sweetened naturally with dates and applesauce, two of nature's natural sweeteners!

Ingredients

15 dates, finely chopped

1¼ cups / 300 ml whole wheat flour

½ cup / 120 ml cocoa powder

2 Tbsp / 30 ml chia seeds

1 tsp / 5 ml baking soda

1 tsp / 5 ml baking powder

½ tsp / 2.5 ml sea salt

2 egg whites

½ cup / 120 ml unsweetened applesauce

½ cup / 120 ml low-fat buttermilk

3 Tbsp / 45 ml honey

1 tsp / 5 ml real vanilla

1 cup / 240 ml steaming hot freshly brewed coffee

Note: This dish is a treat and is not part of your 28-day plan to get *Stripped*.

Nutritional Value Per Serving:

Calories: 99 | Calories from Fat: 11 | Protein: 3.4 g | Carbs: 21 g | Total Fat: 1 g | Saturated Fat: 0 g | Trans Fat: 0 g | Fiber: 4 g | Sodium: 163 mg | Cholesterol: 0 mg | Sugar: 10 g

Method

1 Preheat oven to 350°F / 175°C. Place 14 cupcake liners in muffin tins and place tins on a baking sheet.

2 In a food processor, pulse dates until they are finely chopped and start to come together into a ball. Set aside.

3 In a large bowl, whisk together flour, cocoa powder, chia seeds, baking soda, baking powder and salt until thoroughly combined.

4 Add egg whites, applesauce, buttermilk, honey, vanilla and reserved chopped dates. Whisk together until combined and dates are well distributed. Add hot coffee and carefully whisk until thoroughly combined. Batter will be thin.

5 Fill cupcake liners three-quarters full with batter. Bake for 25 to 30 minutes or until a wooden tooth-pick inserted in center of one cupcake comes out mostly clean. Let stand five minutes then remove cupcakes to a wire rack to cool.

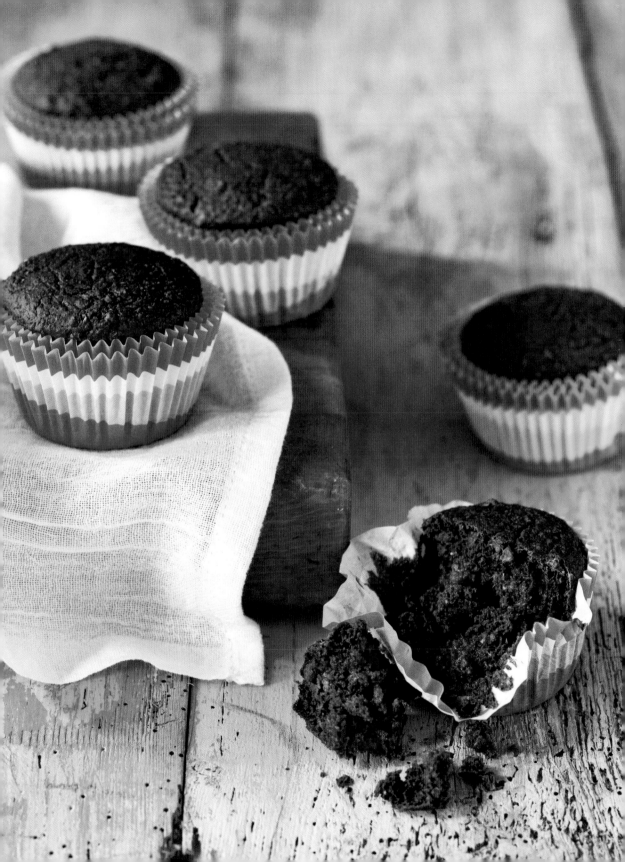

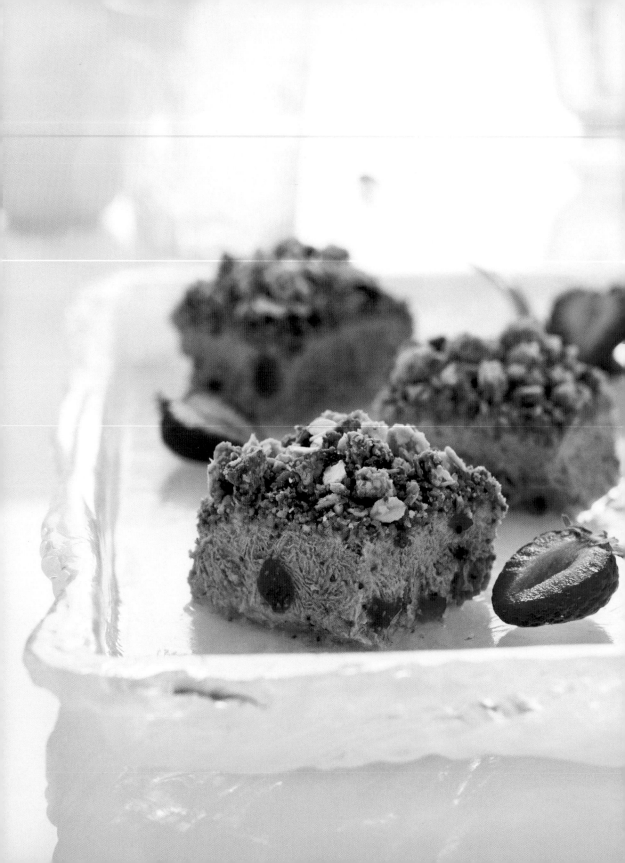

Strawberry Dreamboat Bars ⭑

16 servings

PREP: 15 minutes

TOTAL: 30 minutes

Using fresh strawberries will make this sweet treat perfect for a late-summer BBQ. That being said, you can make it any time of year by using frozen berries – just make sure to slightly thaw them before you begin.

Ingredients

TOPPING:
¼ cup / 60 ml pitted dates, packed
1 Tbsp / 15 ml virgin unrefined coconut oil, softened
2 Tbsp / 30 ml honey
½ cup / 120 ml walnuts
¼ cup / 60 ml whole wheat flour
¼ cup / 60 ml oats
¼ tsp / 1.25 ml sea salt

STRAWBERRY FILLING:
1 x 12.3-oz package Silken firm tofu, drained (must be Silken)
1 cup / 240 ml plain low-fat yogurt
3 Tbsp / 45 ml honey
Juice of 1 lemon (2 to 3 Tbsp / 30 to 45 ml)
1 tsp / 5 ml pure vanilla extract
3 cups / 720 ml fresh or frozen strawberries, divided

Note: This dish is a treat and is not part of your 28-day plan to get *Stripped*.

Nutritional Value Per Serving:

Calories: 94 | Calories from Fat: 30 | Protein: 3 g | Carbs: 14 g | Total Fat: 3 g | Saturated Fat: 1 g | Trans Fat: 0 g | Fiber: 1.4 g | Sodium: 53 mg | Cholesterol: 0 mg | Sugar: 9 g

Method

1 Preheat oven to 350°F / 175°C. In a food processor, add dates, coconut oil and honey, and blend until dates are finely chopped. Add walnuts, flour, oats and salt, and pulse a few times until walnuts are roughly chopped and ingredients are combined. Mixture will be chunky. Pour mixture onto a baking sheet, spread out evenly, and bake in oven until golden brown, stirring once or twice, about 15 minutes. Remove and set aside to cool.

2 In a food processor, blend tofu, yogurt, honey, lemon juice, vanilla and 1½ cups / 360 ml strawberries until smooth. Add remaining strawberries and pulse until roughly chopped. Pour strawberry mixture into a 9 x 9-inch pan and top with walnut mixture.

3 Cover tightly and freeze for at least four hours before serving. Cut into 16 squares and serve. Freeze leftover portions.

Go Bananas Chocolate Tofu Pudding

4 servings
(½ cup / 120 ml per serving)

PREP: 10 minutes

TOTAL: 10 minutes

This dessert is light, cool and creamy – perfect for when you get that craving for chocolate. It's also vegan and proof-on-a-plate that desserts don't need added sugar to be sweet.

Ingredients

¼ cup / 60 ml unsweetened almond milk

3 Tbsp / 45 ml cocoa powder

1 x 12.3-oz box Silken Lite Firm Tofu (must be Silken)

½ tsp / 2.5 ml real vanilla extract

2 very ripe bananas (thaw slightly if using frozen bananas)

scant pinch sea salt

Note: If you want something sweet at the end of the day, make this pudding for your sixth meal as a treat (not every day). It's got protein from the tofu and starchy complex carbs from the banana — a perfect chocolatey Clean meal.

Nutritional Value Per Serving:

Calories: 95 | Calories from Fat: 12 | Protein: 6.5 g | Carbs: 17 g | Total Fat: 1 g | Saturated Fat: 0 g | Trans Fat: 0 g | Fiber: 3 g | Sodium: 164 mg | Cholesterol: 0 mg | Sugar: 7 g

Method

1 Heat almond milk in a small saucepan over medium-high heat until hot. Whisk in cocoa powder until combined.

2 In a blender, add tofu, vanilla, bananas, cocoa mixture and salt. Blend until smooth, stopping to scrape down sides of blender once or twice.

3 Chill in refrigerator for at least 30 minutes; serve.

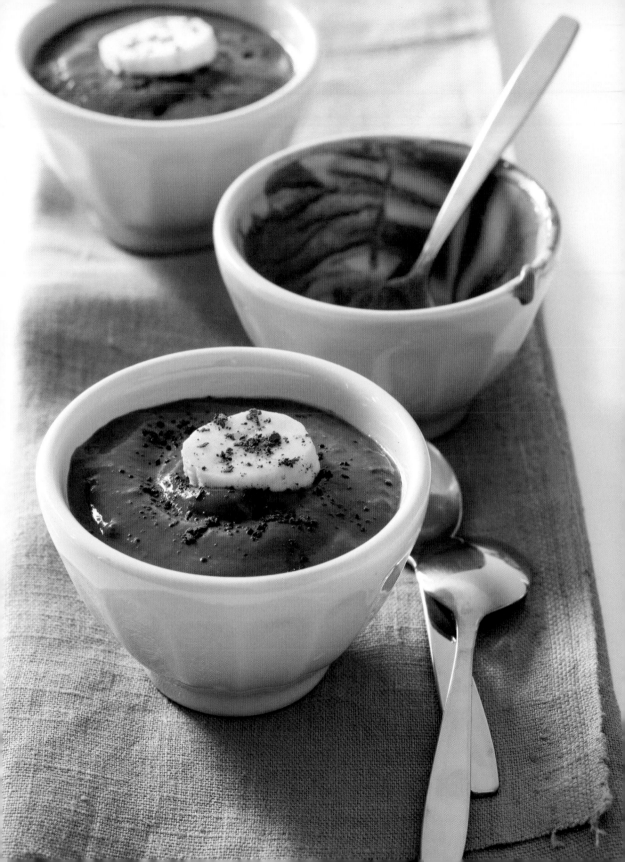

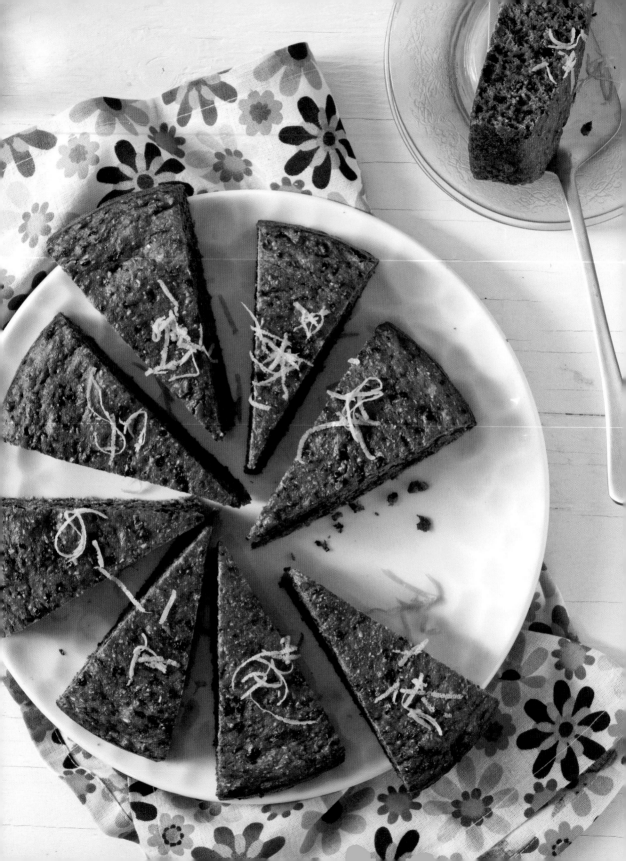

Young at Heart Buttermilk Prune Cake ⭐

12 servings

PREP: 15 minutes

TOTAL: 45 minutes

Don't be fooled by the title – this recipe for Buttermilk Prune Cake is a lot tastier than it sounds. And it's not just for the elderly, despite what you may have heard about prunes in the past! Yes, prunes are high in fiber, but they also increase one's vitality and help slow the aging process of the brain and body. I'll definitely have a slice!

Ingredients

Eat-Clean Cooking Spray
  (see page 214 for recipe)

1 ⅓ cups / 320 ml whole wheat flour

½ tsp / 2.5 ml baking powder

½ tsp / 2.5 ml baking soda

½ tsp / 2.5 ml cinnamon

½ tsp / 2.5 ml nutmeg

¼ tsp / 1.25 ml allspice

½ tsp / 2.5 ml kosher salt

½ cup / 120 ml unsweetened pitted medjool dates

1 cup / 240 ml pitted prunes

½ cup / 120 ml unsweetened applesauce

⅔ cup / 160 ml cultured low-fat buttermilk

3 egg whites

1 Tbsp / 15 ml virgin coconut oil, melted

1 Tbsp / 15 ml orange zest

Note: This dish is a treat and is not part of your 28-day plan to get *Stripped*.

Nutritional Value Per Serving:

Calories: 126 | Calories from Fat: 14 | Protein: 4 g | Carbs: 27 g | Total Fat: 1.6 g | Saturated Fat: 1 g | Trans Fat: 0 g | Fiber: 3 g | Sodium: 145 mg | Cholesterol: 0 mg | Sugar: 12 g

Method

1 Preheat oven to 350°F / 175°C. Spray a 9-inch round cake pan with Eat-Clean Cooking Spray and dust with whole wheat flour.

2 In a large bowl, whisk together all dry ingredients. In a food processor, pulse dates and prunes until finely chopped. Add to dry ingredients. Stir in applesauce, buttermilk, egg whites, coconut oil and orange zest.

3 Pour into prepared cake pan and bake in oven 30 minutes, or until toothpick inserted into center comes out clean. Let cool 10 minutes and remove cake from pan to a wire rack to finish cooling. Cut into 12 slices and enjoy!

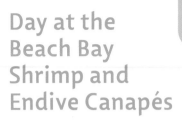

2 servings
PREP: 5 minutes
TOTAL: 5 minutes

Day at the Beach Bay Shrimp and Endive Canapés

Canapés are hors d'oeuvres typically made with a base of bread or crackers and topped with a variety of savory toppings. By swapping the starchy carbs for crisp endive spears, you get a result that maintains the crunch you love without weighing you down.

Ingredients

2 heads Belgian endive

¼ lb / 113.5 g bay shrimp

1 tsp / 5 ml finely chopped fresh tarragon

1 tsp / 5 ml finely chopped fresh chives

Juice of ½ fresh lemon
(1 to 2 Tbsp / 15 to 30 ml)

⅛ tsp / pinch sea salt

⅛ tsp / pinch freshly ground black pepper

Nutritional Value Per Serving:

Calories: 152 | Calories from Fat: 18 |
Protein: 17.5 g | Carbs: 19 g |
Total Fat: 1.7 g | Saturated Fat: 0.01 g |
Trans Fat: 0 g | Fiber: 16 g |
Sodium: 337 mg | Cholesterol: 86 mg |
Sugar: 1.3 g

Method

1 Trim the stalk end of each endive just enough to release outer leaves. Repeat trimming ends and peeling leaves until all larger outer leaves are removed.

2 In a small bowl, combine bay shrimp, tarragon, chives and lemon juice. Season with salt and pepper and toss to combine.

3 Spoon shrimp mixture onto endive spears and serve.

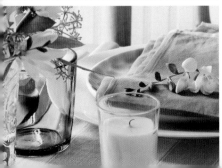

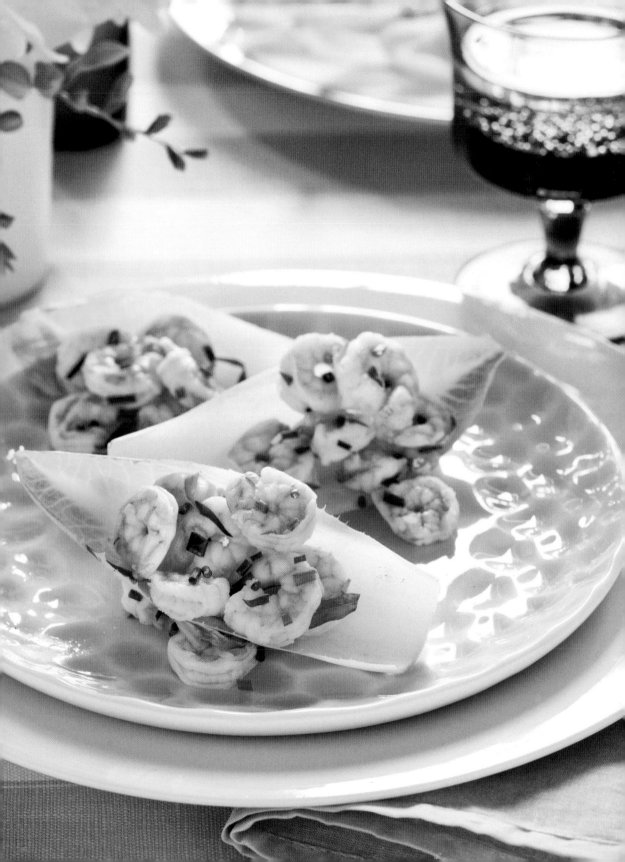

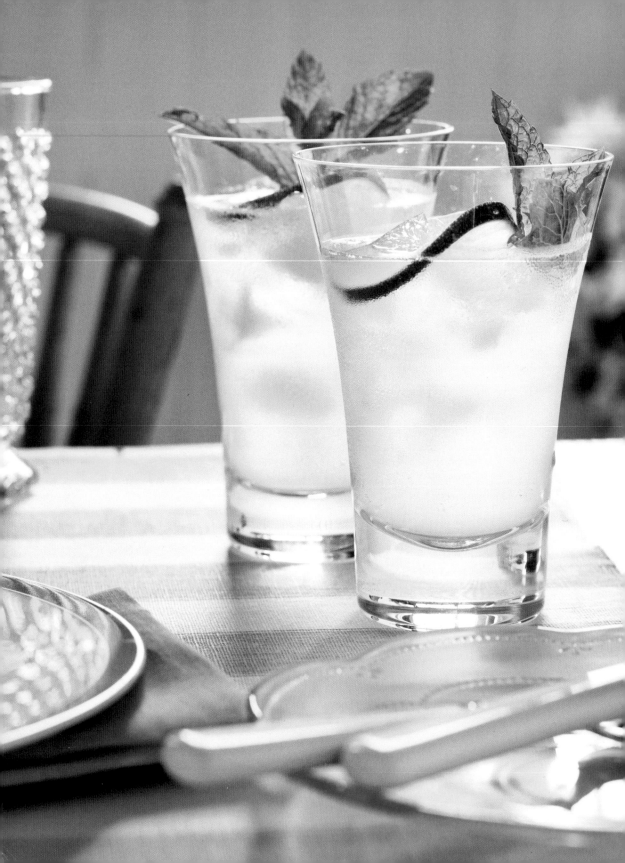

Kombucha Piña Colada (Mocktail)

2 servings
(¾ cup / 180 ml per serving)

PREP: 5 minutes

TOTAL: 5 minutes

Kombucha is a handmade Chinese tea that is delicately cultured for 30 days or longer. During this time, essential nutrients form and combine to create an elixir that immediately works with your body to restore balance and vitality. Kombucha is believed to support: digestion, metabolism, immune system, appetite control, weight control, liver function, body alkalinity, anti-aging, cell integrity and healthy skin and hair.

Ingredients

10 mint leaves

Ice

½ cup / 120 ml organic, unsweetened raw multi-green Kombucha✱

½ cup / 120 ml unsweetened coconut water✱ (not milk)

½ cup / 120 ml 100% pure, unsweetened pineapple juice (not from concentrate)

2 tsp / 10 ml freshly squeezed lime juice

2 lime slices, to garnish

2 sprigs mint, to garnish

✱ You can purchase Kombucha and coconut water at most health food stores.

Nutritional Value Per Serving:

Calories: 53 | Calories from Fat: 2 | Protein: 0.6 g | Carbs: 12 g | Total Fat: 0 g | Saturated Fat: 0 g | Trans Fat: 0 g | Fiber: 0.6 g | Sodium: 68 mg | Cholesterol: 0 mg | Sugar: 8.6 g

Method

1 Add mint leaves and ice to a cocktail shaker. Using the handle of a wooden spoon, muddle the mint until slightly broken apart.

2 Add Kombucha, coconut water, pineapple juice and lime juice. Cover tightly and shake vigorously for 10 seconds until well mixed.

3 Strain mixture into two tall glasses filled with ice. Garnish with lime slices and mint sprigs.

My Heart Sings for You Halibut for Two in Basil-Mint Coconut Broth

2 servings

PREP: 15 minutes

TOTAL: 33 minutes

The title of this recipe may suggest that it's complicated to make but nothing could be further from the truth! Wow your honey on date night with this simple fish recipe. The sauce is sweet and savory – a combination that's sure to inspire a little after-dinner romance.

Ingredients

Eat-Clean Cooking Spray (see page 214 for recipe)

1 leek, white and light green parts only, cleaned and thinly sliced into half moons

1 carrot, peeled and cut into matchsticks

1 parsnip, peeled and cut into matchsticks

Sea salt and freshly ground black pepper, to taste

1 clove garlic, minced

1 cup / 240 ml reduced-fat "lite" coconut milk

1½ cups / 360 ml low-sodium chicken broth

2 sprigs fresh basil

2 sprigs fresh mint

1 lb / 454 g wild-caught halibut fillet, skin removed

Fresh lime wedges, to garnish

Nutritional Value Per Serving:

Calories: 457 | Calories from Fat: 126 | Protein: 50 g | Carbs: 26 g | Total Fat: 14 g | Saturated Fat: 6.8 g | Trans Fat: 0 g | Fiber: 5 g | Sodium: 645 mg | Cholesterol: 76 mg | Sugar: 9 g

Method

1. Coat a large skillet with Eat-Clean Cooking Spray and heat over medium heat. Add leek, carrot and parsnip, and season with salt and pepper. Cook vegetables, stirring occasionally, until they begin to soften without turning brown, about three minutes. Stir in garlic and cook for one minute longer.

2. Stir in coconut milk, broth, basil and mint. Season both sides of halibut with salt and pepper, and gently place halibut in broth. Bring liquid to a simmer, cover skillet leaving a bit of room for steam to escape, and cook fish until opaque in the middle, about 10 minutes.

3. Using a slotted spatula, gently remove fish to a plate and cover with aluminum foil to keep warm.

4. Increase heat under the skillet and boil cooking liquid until slightly reduced, about five minutes. Taste and make any final adjustments to seasoning with salt and pepper.

5. To serve, cut halibut into two pieces and place in two shallow bowls. Divide broth and vegetables evenly into each bowl, discarding any herbs. Serve with fresh lime wedges.

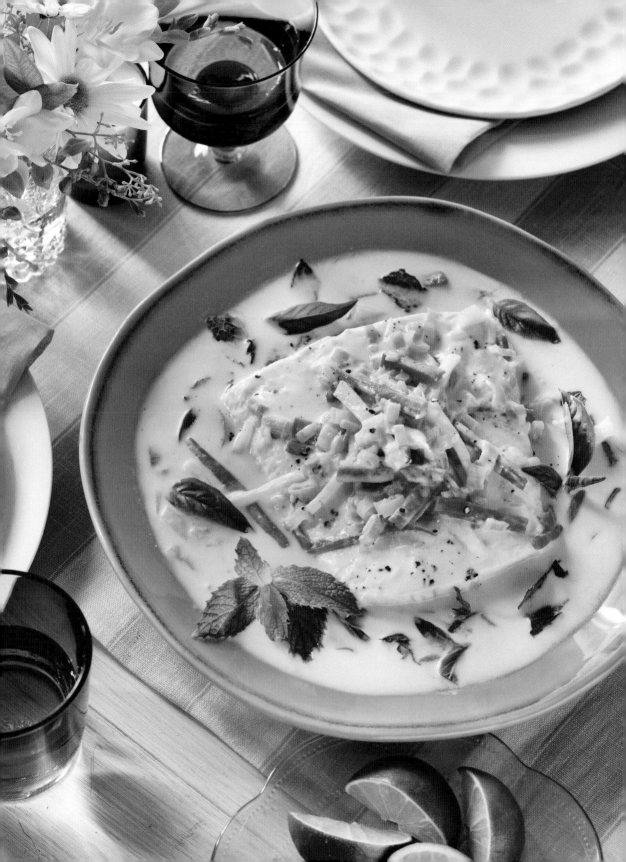

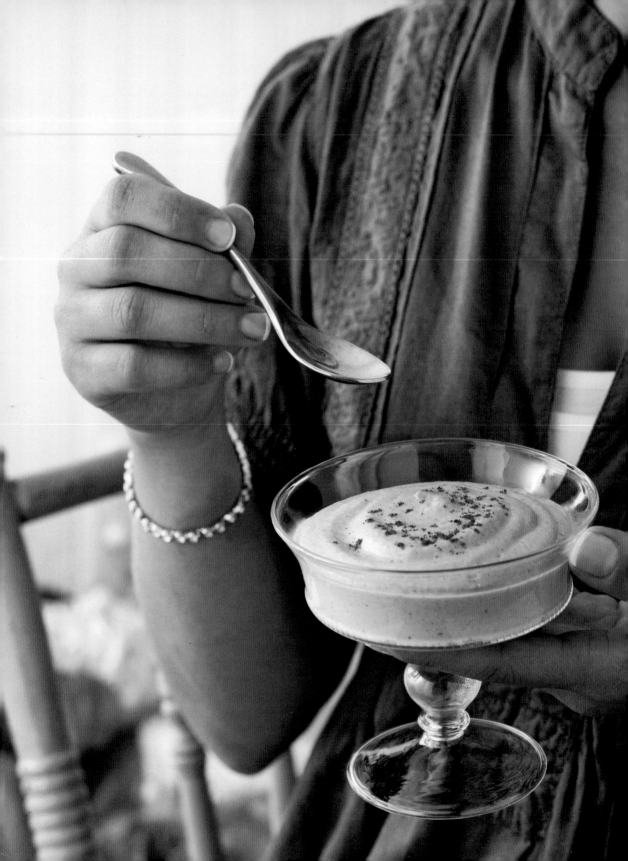

No-Bake Pumpkin Cheesecake Mousse ⍟

4 servings
(1 cup / 240 ml per serving)

PREP: 10 minutes

TOTAL: 10 minutes

When I was a girl the only pumpkin food I knew of was pumpkin pie at Thanksgiving. Now pumpkin products and flavors are popping up everywhere, from tea to scones to yogurt! Here's a deliciously decadent Pumpkin Cheesecake Mousse to satisfy your fall craving for this great gourd.

Ingredients

1 x 12.3-oz package silken firm tofu, drained (must be silken)

1 cup / 240 ml Yogurt Cheese (recipe below)

1 cup / 240 ml unsweetened pumpkin purée (not pumpkin pie mix)

1 Tbsp / 15 ml fresh lemon juice

2 Tbsp / 30 ml honey

½ tsp / 2.5 ml unsulfured blackstrap molasses

1 tsp / 5 ml real vanilla

¼ tsp / 1.25 ml ground cinnamon

⅛ tsp / pinch freshly grated nutmeg

⅛ tsp / pinch ground cloves

⅛ tsp / pinch powdered ginger

Note: This dish is a treat and is not part of your 28-day plan to get *Stripped*.

Nutritional Value Per Serving:

Calories: 145 | Calories from Fat: 20 | Protein: 11.5 g | Carbs: 18 g | Total Fat: 2.5 g | Saturated Fat: 0 g | Trans Fat: 0 g | Fiber: 2 g | Sodium: 63 mg | Cholesterol: 0 mg | Sugar: 12.6 g

Method

1   Add all ingredients to a food processor and blend until combined and very smooth.

2   Chill for one hour before serving.

Yogurt Cheese

Ingredients

2 quarts / 1.9 L low-fat plain yogurt, dairy or soy based

Method

1   Place four layers of damp cheesecloth in a fine mesh sieve or colander. Place the colander over a bowl.

2   Add yogurt and let it drain overnight in the refrigerator.

3   Discard the water from the bowl.

FRONT/BACK COVER PHOTO

BUCETA, PAUL: Hair and makeup by Valeria Nova Styling by Rachel Burton

OTHER PHOTOS

BUCETA, PAUL: Pages 7 (hair / makeup by Valeria Nova, Styling by Rachel Burton),
12 (*Oxygen* cover, model: Lindsay Messina), 26 (hair / makeup by Valeria
Nova, Styling by Nadia Pizziment), 30 (hair / makeup by Valeria Nova,
Styling by Nadia Pizziment), 41 & 115 (*The Eat-Clean Diet: Wokrout
Journal* cover - hair / makeup Lori Fabrizio), 41 (*The Eat-Clean Diet:
Compnaion* cover - hair / makeup Franca Tarullo), 45 (hair / makeup
by Valeria Nova, Styling by Nadia Pizziment), 56 (hair / makeup by
Valeria Nova, Styling by Nadia Pizziment), 62 (hair / makeup by Valeria
Nova, Styling by Nadia Pizziment), 67 (hair / makeup by Valeria Nova,
Styling by Rachel Burton), 86 (hair / makeup by Valeria Nova, Styling by
Rachel Burton), 104 (hair / makeup by Valeria Nova, Styling by Nadia
Pizziment), 110 (hair/makeup by Valeria Nova, Styling by Kiersten
Corradetti), 117 (hair / makeup by Valeria Nova, Styling by Rachel
Burton), 125-137 (hair / makeup by Valeria Nova, Styling by Kiersten
Corradetti) , 138-139 (hair / makeup by Valeria Nova, Styling by Nadia
Pizziment), 153 & 189 (*The Eat-Clean Diet: Recharged!* cover - hair /
makeup by Valeria Nova), 157 (hair / makeup by Valeria Nova,
Styling by Gabriella Caruso Marques), 162 (hair / makeup by Valeria
Nova, Styling by Rachel Burton), 171 (hair / makeup by Valeria Nova,
Styling by Nadia Pizziment), 179 (hair / makeup by Valeria Nova,
Styling by Rachel Burton), 197 (hair / makeup by Valeria Nova,
Styling by Nadia Pizziment).

GRIFFITH, DONNA: Pages 5, 198-301

Food styling by Claire Stubbs

Props provided by Laura Branson, The Prop Room, Robert Kennedy
Publishing, Donna Griffith and Claire Stubbs.

Maya Visnyei - hand model

KENNEDY, ROBERT: 42 & 113

WOLFGANG KALS: Page 110 - Artwork: Lady Gaga - oenogallery.com

Pages 125-131 - Gym routine clothing courtesy of
ELISABETTA ROGIANI · www.rogiani.com

ALL OTHER PHOTOS: istockphoto.com

ACKNOWLEDGMENTS

The entire book-publishing department at Robert Kennedy Publishing needs to be acknowledged.

Wendy Morley, my Book Department Director extraordinaire. Thank you for dedicating yourself to yet another book in the series. You have been there from the start and we have a long way to go yet! You are the best.

Vinita Persaud, my Managing Online Editor who supports the words we print on paper with words and images online. You carry us into the virtual world for others to enjoy. Thank you.

Cali Hoffman, my Production Editor who catches the bloopers and makes my hen scratching sound so much better. Love your style and your ongoing assistance with all things book related.

Meredith Barrett, my Editorial Assistant and Online Editor who performs a myriad of obvious and not so obvious tasks. Thank you for keeping us all straight.

Tara Kher, my Editorial Assistant who handled most of my day-to-day responsibilities while I concentrated on the book. Thanks Tara.

Sharlene Liladhar, my Administrative and Editorial Assistant who also helped handle the multitude of tasks – the biggest of which includes organizing my schedule – so I could keep my life straight and make my deadline. Thank you.

Kiersten Corradetti, my daughter and Online Editor who interfaces with all of you in her passionate and genuine way. Readers, fans, Sisters in Speed and Sisters in Iron – they love you and I love you too.

Rachel Corradetti, another of my daughters who contributes her formidable knowledge (she is studying to be a Naturopathic Doctor) to the table. Thank you and I love you.

Kelsey-Lynn Corradetti, yes another daughter, who styled the recipes and created gorgeous backdrops with her own talented hands. Thank you for your vision and I love you.

Chelsea Kennedy, my wonderful daughter who looked on and laughed when the Corradetti/Kennedy household was caught up in the whirl of hitting book deadlines. I thank you for your wonderful sense of humor. I love you.

Gabriella Caruso, my Art Director and artistic visionary who imagines and creates with brilliance the work you hold in your hands. Thank you and you are amazing.

Jessica Pensabene, my Assistant Art Director whose artistic and creative talents help to make all of the *Eat-Clean Diet* books so popular. Thank you.

Brian Ross and Ellie Jeon, my Editorial Designers whose talented, creative hands make my words come alive on the page. Your energy and vision is wonderful. I thank you.

Donna Griffith and Claire Stubbs, I thank you for your skill at working with light and food, bringing my books to a whole new level. Love your photographic work and food design and love you too. Donna's assistant, Maya Visnyei, helped the days go smoothly and even donated her modeling abilities when necessary. Thank you.

Kiersten Buchner, my Recipe Developer, I thank you for your fierce talent. I knew I was hooked on you that day in Portland when you opened your suitcase! I saw you there. Thank you.

Robert Kennedy, our fearless leader at Robert Kennedy Publishing, who saw an idea six years ago and breathed life into it. I thank God for engineering our meeting those years ago on a Georgetown playground. I love you.

PREVIEW ALL BOOKS IN THE EAT-CLEAN DIET® SERIES AT EATCLEANDIET.COM/BOOKS

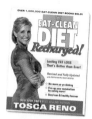

The Eat-Clean Diet Recharged!

The world of weight loss changed forever when *The Eat-Clean Diet* burst on the scene in January 2007. Updated and revised, *The Eat-Clean Diet Recharged!* contains all the facts from the original version, plus in-depth information on staying motivated, living a happier and more productive life, starting an exercise program, how to deal with cellulite and saggy skin, and how to Eat Clean anywhere from parties to restaurants to on the road. Bonus! 50 brand new recipes, with standard, vegan and gluten-free meal plans to accommodate different lifestyles.

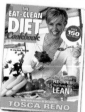

The Eat-Clean Diet Cookbook

A perfect follow-up, this best-selling cookbook is bound to be your go-to guide for Clean meals, with over 150 recipes and gorgeous color photos throughout. From soups and sauces to main courses and desserts, Tosca touches on every food group, combining them into easy-to-prepare, delicious meals that are crowd favorites. Bonus info pages explain the Eat-Clean Principles, protein facts, sugar substitutes and more. Grab your apron and heat up the oven because delicious, healthy food is on the menu tonight!

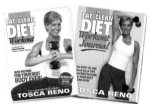

The Eat-Clean Diet Workout & Workout Journal

Eating Clean is a big part of the puzzle, but exercise is the missing piece. In *The Eat-Clean Diet Workout*, Tosca shares her wealth of fitness knowledge with you, including her own workout routines and tips from the best in the business. Bonus 30-minute DVD! Make the most of your workouts by writing them down in *The Eat-Clean Diet Workout Journal*. With space to record your reps, sets, weights, exercises, cardio and goals, you have everything you need to get in your best shape ever.

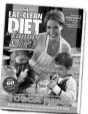

The Eat-Clean Diet for Family & Kids

Tosca Reno has changed the face of health, diet and fitness with her Eat-Clean revolution, and now she's delivering that message to the family. In her foreword, cosmetics icon, CEO and mother-of-three Bobbi Brown says, "Tosca Reno's newest book could not have come at a better time ... Healthy eating needs to start at home and it is our obligation as parents to set the right example for our kids." With tons of tips, tricks and advice, in addition to 60 kid-friendly recipes, this book is sure to become your biggest resource.

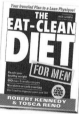

The Eat-Clean Diet for Men

When men saw the results their wives and girlfriends were getting with *The Eat-Clean Diet*, they wanted to know if they could Eat Clean too. The answer? A resounding yes! In fact, Eating Clean was originally developed by, and for, men. So when men Eat Clean they are assured of getting the foods they love, and in quantities that feed their manly muscles. Along with her husband Robert Kennedy, Tosca Reno shows men the way to take care of their specific health problems and their sexual health while creating their optimal physiques. The best news? They never have to count calories or eat like rabbits while doing so.

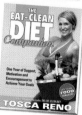

The Eat-Clean Diet Companion

The Eat-Clean Diet Companion is the friendly support you need to make a lifestyle change and lose that extra fat for good. This food journal, personal motivator and resource tool in one contains space to track your Eat-Clean meals and goals, as well as convenient shopping lists, inspirational quotes and photos and food tips from Tosca herself. It's a proven fact that keeping a written log of what you eat can help you make positive changes to your diet, so take control of your life and start today.

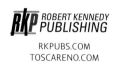

RKP ROBERT KENNEDY PUBLISHING

RKPUBS.COM
TOSCARENO.COM